Contributors

Silvia Ajossa, MD
Department of Obstetrics and Gynecology
Policlinico Universitario di Monserrato
Azienda Ospedaliero Universitaria di
    Cagliari
University of Cagliari
Cagliari, Italy

Juan Luis Alcázar, MD, PhD
Department of Gynecology and Obstetrics
    Medical School
University of Navarra
Pamplona, Spain

Jean L. Browne, MD
Department of Obstetrics, Gynecology,
    and Reproduction
Hospital Universitari Dexeus
Barcelona, Spain

Betlem Graupera, MD, PhD
Department of Obstetrics, Gynecology,
    and Reproduction
Hospital Universitari Dexeus
Barcelona, Spain

Stefano Guerriero, MD, PhD
Department of Obstetrics and
    Gynecology
Policlinico Universitario Duilio Casula
University of Cagliari
Monserrato, Cagliari, Italy

Valerio Mais, MD, PhD
Department of Obstetrics and Gynecology
Policlinico Universitario di Monserrato
Azienda Ospedaliero Universitaria di
    Cagliari
University of Cagliari
Cagliari, Italy

Eleonora Musa, MD
Department of Obstetrics and Gynecology
Policlinico Universitario di Monserrato
Azienda Ospedaliero Universitaria di
    Cagliari
University of Cagliari
Cagliari, Italy

Anna Maria Paoletti, MD, PhD
Department of Obstetrics and Gynecology
Policlinico Universitario di Monserrato
Azienda Ospedaliero Universitaria di
    Cagliari
University of Cagliari
Cagliari, Italy

María Ángela Pascual, MD, PhD
Department of Obstetrics, Gynecology,
    and Reproduction
Hospital Universitari Dexeus
Barcelona, Spain

Alba Piras, MD
Department of Obstetrics and Gynecology
Policlinico Universitario di Monserrato
Azienda Ospedaliero Universitaria di
  Cagliari
University of Cagliari
Cagliari, Italy

Virginia Zanda, MD
Department of Obstetrics and Gynecology
Policlinico Universitario di Monserrato
Azienda Ospedaliero Universitaria di
  Cagliari
University of Cagliari
Cagliari, Italy

Ultrasound of Pelvic Pain in the Non-Pregnant Female

Edited by

Juan Luis Alcázar, MD, PhD
Co-Chairman and Professor
Department of Gynecology and Obstetrics
Medical School, University of Navarra
Pamplona, Spain

María Ángela Pascual, MD, PhD
Head
Gynecological Diagnostic Imaging Unit
Department of Obstetrics, Gynecology, and Reproduction
Hospital Universitari Dexeus
Barcelona, Spain

Stefano Guerriero, MD, PhD
Professor
Department of Obstetrics and Gynecology
Policlinico Universitario Duilio Casula
University of Cagliari
Monserrato, Cagliari, Italy

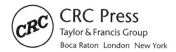

CRC Press
Taylor & Francis Group
Boca Raton London New York

CRC Press is an imprint of the
Taylor & Francis Group, an **informa** business

CRC Press
Taylor & Francis Group
6000 Broken Sound Parkway NW, Suite 300
Boca Raton, FL 33487-2742

© 2019 by Taylor & Francis Group, LLC
CRC Press is an imprint of Taylor & Francis Group, an Informa business

No claim to original U.S. Government works

Printed on acid-free paper

International Standard Book Number-13: 978-0-8153-6499-3 (Hardback)
978-0-8153-6497-9 (Paperback)

Visit the Taylor & Francis Web site at
http://www.taylorandfrancis.com

and the CRC Press Web site at
http://www.crcpress.com

Contents

CHAPTER 1

Benign Adnexal Masses and Adnexal Torsion

Juan Luis Alcázar

INTRODUCTION

Adnexal masses are relatively common in women. Most of these tumors are benign.[1] Histologically, the ovary may be the origin of many different types of benign tumors and there are tumors arising from the fallopian tube (Table 1.1). Most benign tumors remain asymptomatic but some of them may cause symptoms, such as pelvic/abdominal pain, menstrual disorders, or symptoms related to space-occupying lesions. In fact, adnexal torsion is most frequent in benign tumors than in ovarian cancer.[2] Transvaginal ultrasound has been shown as the best imaging technique for assessing adnexal masses,[3] especially when performed by an expert examiner.[4] In this chapter, we will review the ability of transvaginal ultrasound for discriminating between the most common types of benign lesions arising from de ovary and tube, as well as current management options. We will also address the role of ultrasound in diagnosing and managing adnexal torsion.

BENIGN ADNEXAL MASSES: DIAGNOSIS AND MANAGEMENT

Serous Cystadenoma

Serous cystadenoma constitutes about 25% of all benign epithelial ovarian tumors arising from the ovary; 5% of them are bilateral and most of them appear in the fourth to sixth decades of life.[1] The typical ultrasound appearance of serous cystadenomas is a smooth, thin-walled, anechoic, fluid-filled lesion with a mean size of 5–8 cm (Figure 1.1a).[5,6] Septations may appear in 14% of the cases and irregular wall or even papillary projections may be present in up to 3% of serous cystadenomas (Figure 1.1b).[5] Color score may vary from absent to moderate flow within the cystic wall.

TABLE 1.1   Histologic Classification of Benign Ovarian Tumors

Epithelial tumors
- Serous cystadenoma/cystadenofibroma
- Mucinous cystadenoma/cystadenofibroma
- Endometrioma
- Transitional call tumor (Brenner tumor)

Nonepithelial tumors
- Sex cord–stromal tumors
  - Fibroma/fibrothecoma
  - Sclerosing stromal tumor
  - Thecoma
- Germ-cell tumors
  - Mature cystic teratoma (biphasic/triphasic)
  - Stroma ovarii (monodermal teratoma)

Other rare benign tumors

Mucinous Cystadenomas

Mucinous cystadenomas constitute 25% of all benign epithelial ovarian tumors; 10% of them are bilateral and usually appear in the fifth and sixth decades of life.[1] The typical ultrasound appearance of mucinous cystadenoma is a multilocular smooth cyst with a mean tumor size of 11 cm (range 3–30 cm) (Figure 1.2).[7,8] Color score is usually absent, or scanty and papillary projections may appear in 20% of the cases. Caspi et al. described that the presence of different echogenicity in different locules of the lesion is almost pathognomonic of a mucinous tumor.[9]

Endometrioma

Endometrioma is addressed in detail in another chapter of the book. But know that the typical ultrasound appearance of endometrioma is a unilocular cyst with ground-glass echogenicity (Figure 1.3).[5,6]

Cystadenofibroma

Cystadenofibromas are relatively uncommon epithelial ovarian tumors. The serous type is much more frequent than the mucinous type.[1] The most common finding is a unilocular-solid or multilocular-solid cyst with one or two papillary projections (Figure 1.4).[10]

Brenner Tumor

Benign Brenner tumors or transitional cell tumors constitute about 5% of all epithelial benign tumors. About 7%–8% of them may be bilateral and they usually appear in the fifth or sixth decades of life.[1] Brenner tumors usually appear at ultrasound examination as multilocular-solid or solid adnexal lesions (Figure 1.5).[11] Most cases exhibit no flow or minimal flow at color score assessment, and calcifications may be present in up to 87% of the cases. Tumor mean size is 7 cm.

(a)

(b)

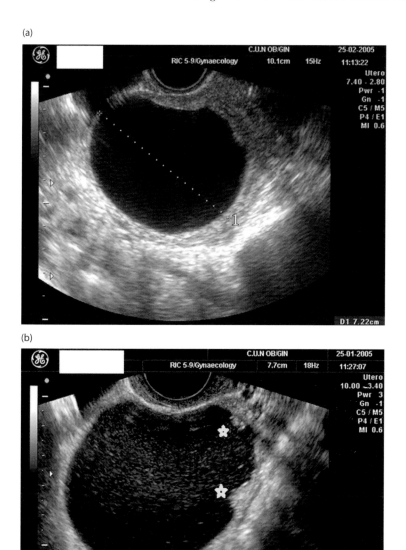

FIGURE 1.1   (a) Transvaginal ultrasound showing a unilocular thin-walled cyst corresponding to a serous cystadenoma. (b) In some cases, wall irregularities (asterisks) may appear.

Mature Teratoma

Mature teratomas are among the most frequent benign ovarian tumors (25%) and the most frequent nonepithelial germ cell derived ovarian tumors (92%).[1] The typical appearance of a mature teratoma is a unilocular cyst with mixed echogenicity due to different cyst's content (bone, hair, fluid, fat) and acoustic shadowing (Figure 1.6).[5,6] Color signals are usually absent. The presence of the so-called Rokitansky nodule is considered as pathognomonic

(a)

(b)

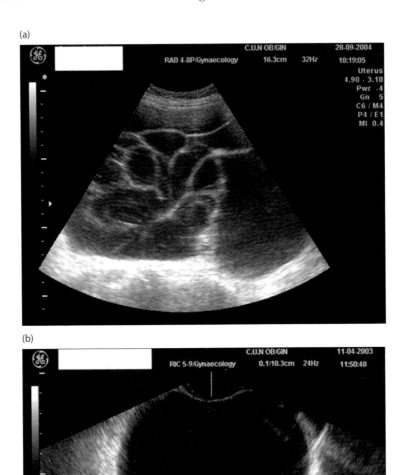

FIGURE 1.2   (a) Transvaginal ultrasound showing a large multilocular cyst, corresponding to a mucinous cystadenoma. (b) In some cases these tumors appear as unilocular cysts with a focal area with multiple small cysts (honeycomb sign) (asterisk).

for mature teratomas (Figure 1.7). This is caused by high-density tissue such as bone, teeth, or floating hair.

A particular type of benign monodermic mature teratoma is the struma ovarii. This tumor is characterized by the presence of thyroid tissue. At ultrasound examination the typical appearance of struma ovarii is a multilocular-solid mass with moderate or abundant color score (Figure 1.8).[12,13]

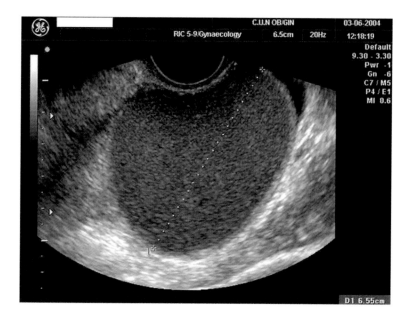

FIGURE 1.3   Transvaginal ultrasound showing the typical appearance of an ovarian endometrioma: Unilocular cyst with ground-glass content.

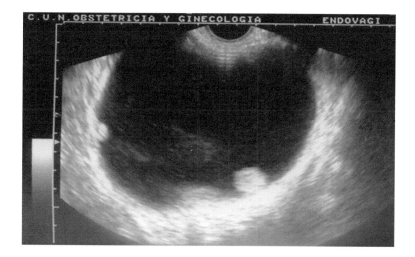

FIGURE 1.4   Transvaginal ultrasound showing a cyst with papillary projections corresponding to a serous cystadenofibroma.

Fibroma/Fibrothecoma

Fibromas are the most common subtype of sex cord–stromal ovarian tumors. They account for 4%–6% of all benign ovarian tumors.[1] They usually appear in peri- and postmenopausal women. The typical ultrasound appearance of ovarian fibromas and fibrothecomas is a well-defined solid mass (Figure 1.9).[14] Mean tumor size is 5–7 cm, and the color score is usually minimal or moderate. Acoustic shadowing appears in one-third of the cases.

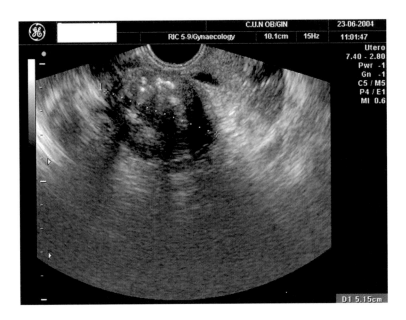

FIGURE 1.5 Transvaginal ultrasound showing a well-defined solid lesion with hyperechoic areas and shadowing corresponding to a benign Brenner tumor.

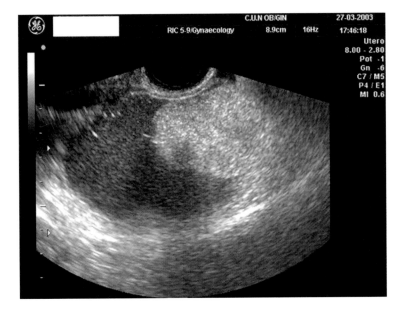

FIGURE 1.6 Transvaginal ultrasound showing a unilocular lesion with mixed echogenicity corresponding to a mature teratoma.

Hydrosalpinx

Hydrosalpinx is related to the obstruction of the fimbrial end of the tube and subsequent filling with fluid, usually as a consequence of pelvic inflammatory disease. The typical ultrasound appearance of hydrosalpinx is an elongated cystic mass with complete and incomplete septations (Figure 1.10a).[5]

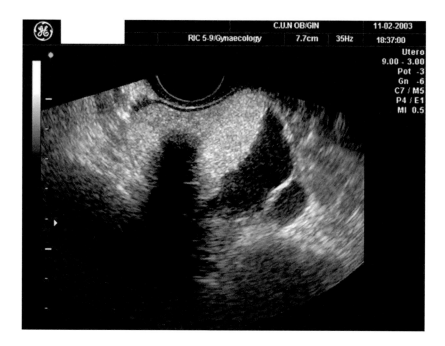

FIGURE 1.7 Another case of ovarian mature teratoma. A unilocular lesion with mixed echogenicity. A shadow due to the presence of the Rokitansky nodule is observed.

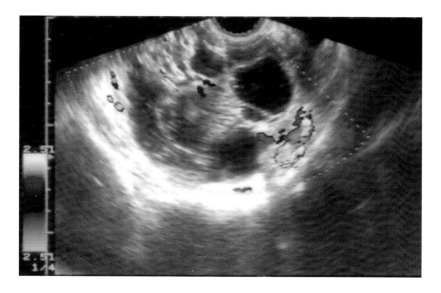

FIGURE 1.8 Transvaginal ultrasound showing a multilocular-solid lesion with abundant vascularization corresponding to a benign struma ovarii.

In some cases the "cogwheel" sign (a sonolucent cogwheel-shaped structure visible in the cross section of the tube with thick wall) and the "beads-on-a-string" sign (hyperechoic mural nodules measuring 2–3 mm visible in a cross section of the tube) can be seen (Figure 1.10b).[15] The role of color Doppler is limited in these lesions.[16]

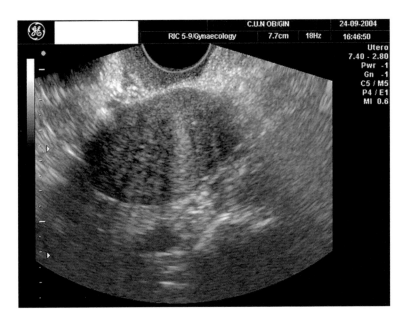

FIGURE 1.9   Transvaginal ultrasound showing a well-defined homogeneous solid lesion with fan-shape shadowing corresponding to an ovarian fibroma.

Paraovarian and Paratubal Cyst

Paraovarian or paratubal cysts arise from the mesosalpinx or the broad ligament close to the ovary or fallopian tube. The typical ultrasound appearance is a unilocular cystic lesion with a mean size of 4 cm that should be identified close to the ipsilateral ovary (Figure 1.11).[17]

Accuracy of Ultrasound for the Specific Diagnosis of Adnexal Masses

According to two of the largest case series to date, the diagnostic performance of ultrasound is high for some of the benign lesions but is poor for some others (Table 1.2).[18,19] A patient's menopausal status may affect this diagnostic performance,[19] decreasing sensitivity for some types of lesions such as endometrioma and hydrosalpinx.

Interestingly, agreement for the typical pattern for serous cystadenoma, endometrioma, and mature teratoma among different observers is good.[20] The use of other imaging techniques such as CT scan or MRI does not improve the overall diagnostic performance of ultrasound.[3,21]

Management of Benign Adnexal Masses

Traditionally, the management of benign persistent adnexal masses has been surgical removal.[22] The currently preferred surgical approach should be laparoscopy.[23,24] Clearly, this management should be considered for symptomatic adnexal masses, but it is also considered for asymptomatic adnexal masses.[22] The main reasons advocated for surgical removal of asymptomatic adnexal masses are fear of complication (torsion, rupture) or malignancy transformation. However, torsion is uncommon[18] and there is no evidence that removing benign adnexal masses decreases the risk of having ovarian cancer.[25]

(a)

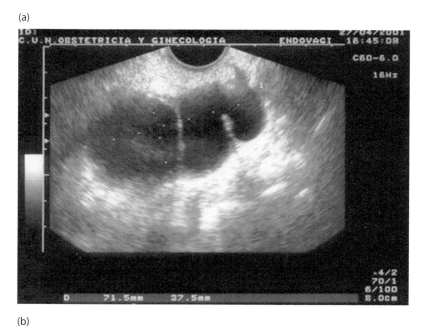

(b)

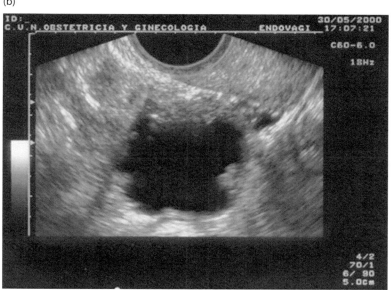

FIGURE 1.10 Transvaginal ultrasound showing the typical findings of hydrosalpinx. (a) An elongated cystic lesion with complete and incomplete septations. (b) A case showing the "beads-on-a-string" sign.

In the last decade, some reports have shown that conservative management with serial follow-up may be an option for asymptomatic adnexal masses. The risk of malignancy for simple cysts in postmenopausal asymptomatic patients is very low (0.19%) and up to 46% of them will resolved spontaneously.[26] Therefore, current management for these type of lesions should be follow-up, even for lesions up to 10 cm in size.[3,27] There is no clear information about frequency of follow-up scans and for how long these lesions should be monitored. A

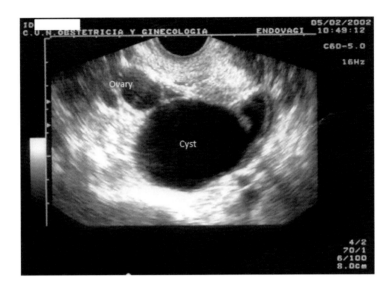

FIGURE 1.11   Transvaginal ultrasound showing the typical appearance of a paraovarian cyst as a unilocular cystic lesion identified close to the ipsilateral ovary.

TABLE 1.2   Prevalence and Diagnostic Performance for Benign Tumors in Two Large Case Series

	Prevalence among Benign Tumors (%)	Sensitivity (%)	Specificity (%)
Serous cyst	18.6–20.0	54.0–82.7	94.0–94.6
Mucinous cyst	6.0–10.7	33.7–36.0	97.0–98.9
Endometrioma	24.9–33.2	77.0–88.4	97.1–98.0
Mature teratoma	14.3–14.5	86.0–86.3	98.5–99.0
Fibroma/fibrothecoma	2.1–2.4	25.0–42.0	99.0–99.8
Brenner	0.3	20	99.8
Cystadenofibroma	2.7–4.9	8.0–26.1	97–98.0
Hydrosalpinx	2.6–3.3	81.8–86.0	98.0–99.8
Paraovarian cyst	2.6–3.2	14.0–58.5	99.0–99.6

Source: Sokalska A et al. *Ultrasound Obstet Gynecol,* 2009;34:462–70; Alcázar JL et al. *Maturitas,* 2011;68:182–8.

yearly scan for 2–5 years, if no change in the lesion occurs, seems to be reasonable.[28,29] This management may also be advised for simple cysts in premenopausal women.[3,28]

Alcázar et al. reported a prospective study in 166 premenopausal asymptomatic women, including 232 benign-appearing adnexal masses.[28] Conservative management with serial follow-up was performed. Median follow-up was 48.5 months (range 6 to 192 months). Ninety-five (40.9%) masses resolved spontaneously with a median elapsed time from diagnosis to resolution of 40 months. There was one case of ovarian torsion (0.4%) and two women developed ovarian cancer (0.8%).

A recent report from the IOTA group comprising more than 5000 women with asymptomatic benign-appearing adnexal masses and managed conservatively with serial follow-up for at least 2 years found that the risk for torsion was 0.4%, the risk for rupture was 0.2%, and the risk for developing a malignancy was 0.8%.[30]

Alcázar et al. also reported on conservative management of benign-appearing solid adnexal masses in asymptomatic postmenopausal women. Criteria for benignity was the presence of a well-defined purely solid lesion with scanty or no color signals.[31] Their study included 99 women and they found that two (2%) developed ovarian cancer. They concluded that conservative management might be an option for these women.

Several studies including small case series have shown that mature cystic teratomas tend to slowly grow (1–1.3 mm per year) during conservative management.[28,32,33] However, follow-up time was short for most of these studies. Pascual et al. followed women with an ultrasound diagnosis of mature teratoma ($n = 408$) with the longest follow-up.[34] They reported that 103 women underwent surgery during follow-up, most of them during the first 5 years after diagnosis. They found one case of ovarian torsion (0.2%) and two borderline ovarian tumors (0.4%). The main reason for surgery in these cases was increased tumor size (growing 4.8 mm/year) of the remaining 278 women who did not undergo surgery, and no significant change in tumor size was observed with a median follow-up time of 45.6 months (range: 6–147 months). Women who did not undergo surgery had smaller lesions at diagnosis, were older, and had bilateral lesions less frequently than those who ultimately underwent surgery. These authors concluded that expectant management might be a reasonable option for benign-appearing mature teratomas in asymptomatic women.

In conclusion, the risk of torsion, rupture, or malignancy in benign-appearing adnexal masses seems to be low. There is growing evidence that conservative management of these lesions in asymptomatic women is a safe option.

ADNEXAL TORSION

Adnexal torsion may affect women of all ages, accounting for about 3% of gynecologic emergencies.[35,36] It refers to a total or partial twist of the ovary around its vascular axis resulting in vascular compromise and ovarian ischemia.[35]

Four pathological patterns have been described: tubo-ovarian torsion, ovarian torsion (Figure 1.12), tubal torsion (Figure 1.13), and mesentero-tubal torsion.[35]

Adnexal torsion may occur in an otherwise normal ovary or tube, but there are some risk factors to take into account such as previous adnexal torsion, ovarian hyperstimulation syndrome, pregnancy, ovarian tumor, polycystic ovary, and previous tubal ligation.[36] It has been shown that adnexal masses larger than >5 cm were at greater risk for torsion.[37] However, this has been challenged by other authors.[38] Endometriomas, tubo-ovarian abscesses, hydrosalpinges, and malignancies are associated with adhesions and rarely are cause of torsion.[36]

When an adnexal mass is present, it has been reported that mature teratoma is the type of tumor most frequently found at surgery.[35] However, it has shown in prospective longitudinal studies to be a very small proportion of teratomas torted.[34]

Clinical signs of adnexal torsion are nonspecific.[35,36] Acute pain, either constant or intermittent, is present in 90% of the cases; nausea (70%), vomiting (45%), and fever may also appear. The intensity of pain varies and it is not always severe. Sometimes the episodes of pain may occur for several days or even months before diagnosis.

The right adnexal is more frequently involved and may mimic appendicitis.

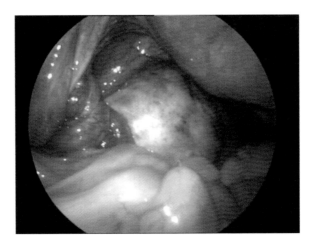

FIGURE 1.12   Laparoscopic image of a torted ovary.

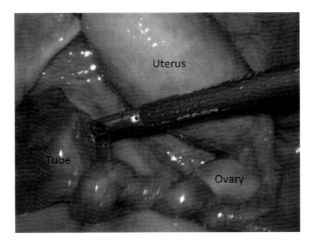

FIGURE 1.13   Laparoscopic image of a torted fallopian tube.

Physical examination has limitations for correct preoperative diagnosis of adnexal torsion, and laboratory tests are nonspecific with slight leukocytosis and elevation of C-reactive protein.[36] Peritonitis is a rare event but may occur in cases of prolonged twisted adnexal.[35]

Emergent laparoscopy is the treatment of choice.[39] Detorsion should be considered always, even in "blue-black" ovaries.

In the case of an adnexal mass, delaying cystectomy may be considered for avoiding additional trauma to the ovary. Oophorectomy or adnexectomy should be considered only in peri- or postmenopausal women. In some cases oophoropexy may be considered, especially when a long ovarian ligament is observed.

Ultrasound Assessment in Adnexal Torsion

Pelvic ultrasound remains as the first imaging technique assessing women with suspected adnexal torsions. It is widely available, relatively inexpensive, and does not use ionizing radiation.[35]

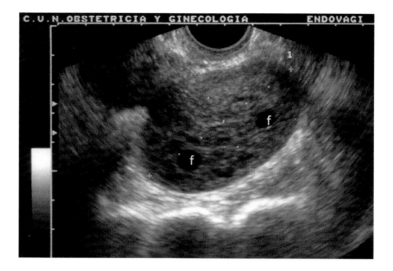

FIGURE 1.14   Transvaginal ultrasound showing an ovarian torsion at early stage. The ovary is an enlarged edema with few and disperse follicles (f).

The most common finding in adnexal torsion as assessed by grayscale ultrasound is the presence of an enlarged ovary with echogenic stromal edema and few follicles peripherally displaced (Figure 1.14).[40] Ovarian size usually exceeds 4 cm. The presence of a fluid-debris level within the follicles has been considered as a pathognomonic sign of ovarian torsion (Figure 1.15).[41] However, this has not been confirmed in a large study.

Another finding associated to ovarian torsion is the presence of the so-called follicular ring sign.[42] This finding is characterized by the presence of a hyperechoic ring surrounding the follicles (Figure 1.16). This finding has been reported in up to 80% of cases.[42]

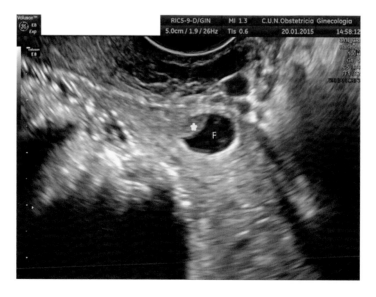

FIGURE 1.15   Transvaginal ultrasound showing an ovarian torsion. In this case, debris (asterisk) within a follicle may be observed (F).

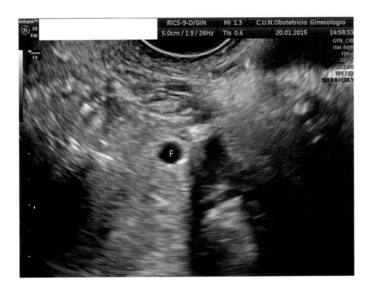

FIGURE 1.16 Transvaginal ultrasound showing an ovarian torsion showing the echogenic rim around the follicle (F).

The presence of an adnexal neoplasia has been reported in 15%–33% of the cases,[43,44] being the most frequent lesion in the mature teratoma.[43] However, other lesions such as serous cysts or hemorrhagic cysts may be present (Figure 1.17).

Free pelvic fluid in the cul-de-sac may be present in 21%–87% of the cases.[40,45,46] However, this is a nonspecific finding.

The twisted pedicle (the "whirlpool sign") can be detected using color Doppler (Figure 1.18) or grayscale ultrasound (Figure 1.19).[47–49] This finding is considered almost pathognomonic for adnexal torsion. When observed, the adnexal torsion was confirmed at laparoscopy in 90%–100% of patients.

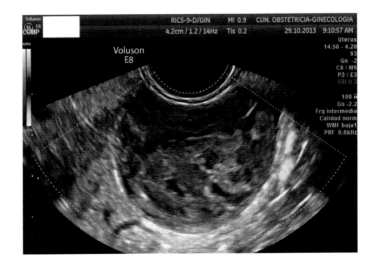

FIGURE 1.17 Transvaginal ultrasound showing an ovarian torsion in a case of a hemorrhagic cyst. No color Doppler signal may be observed in the cyst wall.

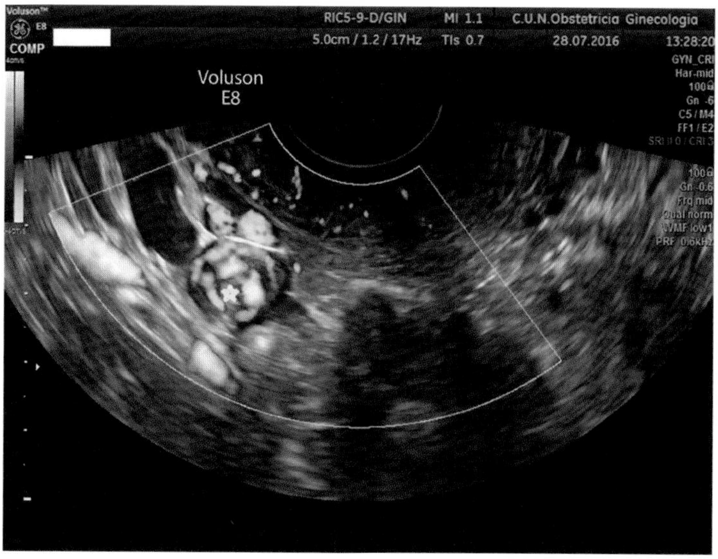

FIGURE 1.18 Transvaginal color ultrasound depicting the whirlpool sign (asterisk) in a case of adnexal torsion.

Smorgik et al. reported that ultrasound findings might vary according to duration of symptoms. They found that enlarged ovaries with peripheral follicles were visible in 100% of women with symptoms lasting less than 24 hours. The "solid"-appearing ovary was never seen in these women. However, 62% of women with symptoms presenting for more than 24 hours had a solid-appearing ovary. In the other group, the presence of pelvic free fluid was also more frequent.[45]

The role of color and pulsed Doppler in the assessment of adnexal torsion is still under debate. Fleischer et al. reported that absence of ovarian stromal venous and arterial flow was associated with necrosis. On the contrary, all viable ovaries had at least ovarian stromal venous flow.[50] However, these findings have not been confirmed in other case series.[51] In fact, normal ovarian blood flow has been reported in up to 40% of surgically confirmed cases of ovarian torsion.[52]

Lee et al. reported that when no flow could be detected within the twisted vascular pedicle, ovaries were necrotic.[47]

The presence of arterial flow within the ovary does not rule out adnexal torsion. Shadinger et al. found that the duration of pain was not associated with the absence or presence of both arterial and venous flow.[46]

Role of Computerized Tomographic Scan (CT Scan) and Magnetic Resonance Imaging (MRI) in Adnexal Torsion

As stated earlier, CT scan and MRI are not the first-line imaging techniques for assessing patients with clinical suspicion of adnexal torsion. However, they may be a problem-solving technique when ultrasound findings are not clear, especially in some clinical scenarios such as pediatric patients and pregnancy.

(a)

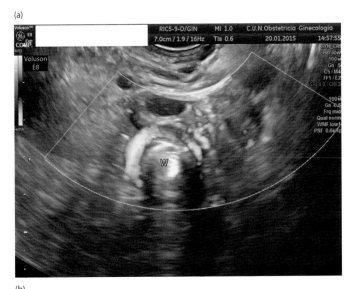

(b)

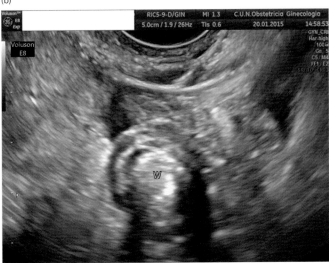

FIGURE 1.19   (a) Transvaginal color ultrasound depicting the whirlpool sign (w) in a case of adnexal torsion. (b) Albeit color Doppler is useful to detect the whirlpool sign, this can also be detected in grayscale ultrasound (w).

Common findings on CT scan are nonspecific, the most common being the displacement of the enlarged adnexal to the midline.[35] When a mass is present, this can be detected by CT scan.[40] Other findings, such as pelvic free fluid, obliteration of fat planes, and ovarian hemorrhage may be observed.[35,40]

In MRI, the edema of the ovary appears as hyperintense on T2-weighted images.[35]

Other Entities That Might Mimic Adnexal Torsion

There are different entities that might mimic adnexal torsion that should be considered within the differential diagnosis. Most of them will be addressed in other chapters of this book and include appendicitis, diverticulitis, ureterolithiasis, pelvic inflammatory disease, hemorrhagic corpus luteum, and ovarian hyperstimulation syndrome.

CONCLUSIONS

Benign ovarian tumors are common in women. Most of them are symptomatic.

Ultrasound is the best imaging technique for assessing benign adnexal masses. Although surgical removal by minimally invasive surgery is still the gold standard management for theses masses, there is growing evidence that conservative management may be a safe option for these cases with a low rate of complications such as torsion, rupture, or malignant transformation.

Ovarian torsion is a clinically relevant emergency in gynecology. Ultrasound should be the first-line imaging technique for evaluating patients suspected of adnexal torsion. There are some ultrasound findings that may contribute significantly to the diagnosis of adnexal torsion, the whirlpool sign being the most specific one. The role of color and pulsed Doppler is controversial. CT scan or MRI may be problem-solving techniques in some cases.

REFERENCES

1. Tavassoli FA, Devilee P, eds. *WHO Gynecological Tumor Classification*. Lyon: IARC Press. 2003.
2. Sommerville M, Grimes DA, Koonings PP, Campbell K. Ovarian neoplasms and the risk of adnexal torsion. *Am J Obstet Gynecol*. 1991;164:577–8.
3. American College of Obstetricians and Gynecologists' Committee on Practice Bulletins—Gynecology. Practice Bulletin No. 174: Evaluation and Management of Adnexal Masses. *Obstet Gynecol*. 2016;128:e210–26.
4. Meys EM, Kaijser J, Kruitwagen RF, Slangen BF, Van Calster B, Aertgeerts B, Verbakel JY, Timmerman D, Van Gorp T. Subjective assessment versus ultrasound models to diagnose ovarian cancer: A systematic review and meta-analysis. *Eur J Cancer*. May 2016;58:17–29.
5. Guerriero S, Ajossa S, Gerada M, Virgilio B, Pilloni M, Galvan R, Laparte C, Melis GB. Transvaginal ultrasound in the diagnosis of extrauterine pelvic diseases. *Expert Rev Obstet Gynecol*. 2008;3:731–52.
6. Sayasneh A, Ekechi C, Ferrara L, Kaijser J, Stalder C, Sur S, Timmerman D, Bourne T. The characteristic ultrasound features of specific types of ovarian pathology (review). *Int J Oncol*. 2015;46:445–58.
7. Pascual MA, Guerriero S, Rams N et al. Clinical and ultrasound features of benign, borderline and invasive mucinous ovarian tumors. *Eur J Gynecol Oncol* 2017;37:382–6.
8. Moro F, Zannoni GF, Arciuolo D, Pasciuto T, Amoroso S, Mascilini F, Mainenti S, Scambia G, Testa AC. Imaging in gynecological disease (11): Clinical and ultrasound features of mucinous ovarian tumors. *Ultrasound Obstet Gynecol*. 2017;50:261–70.
9. Caspi B, Hagay Z, Appelman Z. Variable echogenicity as a sonographic sign in the preoperative diagnosis of ovarian mucinous tumors. *J Ultrasound Med*. 2006;25:1583–5.
10. Alcázar JL, Errasti T, Mínguez JA, Galán MJ, García-Manero M, Ceamanos C. Sonographic features of ovarian cystadenofibromas: Spectrum of findings. *J Ultrasound Med*. 2001;20:915–9.
11. Dierickx I, Valentin L, Van Holsbeke C, Jacomen G, Lissoni AA, Licameli A, Testa A, Bourne T, Timmerman D. Imaging in gynecological disease (7): Clinical and ultrasound features of Brenner tumors of the ovary. *Ultrasound Obstet Gynecol*. 2012;40:706–13.

12. Royo P, Alcázar JL, Virgen M, Mazaira J, Jurado M, Lopez G. B-mode and Doppler features of struma ovarii. *Ultrasound Obstet Gynecol.* 2008;31:109–10.

13. Savelli L, Testa AC, Timmerman D, Paladini D, Ljungberg O, Valentin L. Imaging of gynecological disease (4): Clinical and ultrasound characteristics of struma ovarii. *Ultrasound Obstet Gynecol.* 2008;32:210–9.

14. Paladini D, Testa A, Van Holsbeke C, Mancari R, Timmerman D, Valentin L. Imaging in gynecological disease (5): Clinical and ultrasound characteristics in fibroma and fibrothecoma of the ovary. *Ultrasound Obstet Gynecol.* 2009;34:188–95.

15. Timor-Tritsch IE, Lerner JP, Monteagudo A, Murphy KE, Heller DS. Transvaginal sonographic markers of tubal inflammatory disease. *Ultrasound Obstet Gynecol.* 1998;12:56–66.

16. Guerriero S, Ajossa S, Lai MP, Mais V, Paoletti AM, Melis GB. Transvaginal ultrasonography associated with colour Doppler energy in the diagnosis of hydrosalpinx. *Hum Reprod.* 2000;15:1568–72.

17. Savelli L, Ghi T, De Iaco P, Ceccaroni M, Venturoli S, Cacciatore B. Paraovarian/paratubal cysts: Comparison of transvaginal sonographic and pathological findings to establish diagnostic criteria. *Ultrasound Obstet Gynecol.* 2006;28:330–4.

18. Sokalska A, Timmerman D, Testa AC, Van Holsbeke C, Lissoni AA, Leone FP, Jurkovic D, Valentin L. Diagnostic accuracy of transvaginal ultrasound examination for assigning a specific diagnosis to adnexal masses. *Ultrasound Obstet Gynecol.* 2009;34:462–70.

19. Alcázar JL, Guerriero S, Laparte C, Ajossa S, Ruiz-Zambrana A, Melis GB. Diagnostic performance of transvaginal gray-scale ultrasound for specific diagnosis of benign ovarian cysts in relation to menopausal status. *Maturitas.* 2011;68:182–8.

20. Guerriero S, Alcázar JL, Pascual MA, Ajossa S, Gerada M, Bargellini R, Virgilio B, Melis GB. Diagnosis of the most frequent benign ovarian cysts: Is ultrasonography accurate and reproducible? *J Womens Health (Larchmt).* 2009;18:519–27.

21. Glanc P, Benacerraf B, Bourne T et al. First International Consensus Report on Adnexal Masses: Management recommendations. *J Ultrasound Med.* 2017;36:849–63.

22. RCOG/BSGE. *Management of suspected ovarian masses in premenopausal women (Green-top Guideline No. 62).* November 2011.

23. Medeiros LR, Rosa DD, Bozzetti MC, Fachel JM, Furness S, Garry R, Rosa MI, Stein AT. Laparoscopy versus laparotomy for benign ovarian tumour. *Cochrane Database Syst Rev.* 2009 April 15;(2):CD004751.

24. Canis M, Rabischong B, Houlle C, Botchorishvili R, Jardon K, Safi A, Wattiez A, Mage G, Pouly JL, Bruhat MA. Laparoscopic management of adnexal masses: A gold standard? *Curr Opin Obstet Gynecol.* 2002;14:423–8.

25. Crayford TJ, Campbell S, Bourne TH, Rawson HJ, Collins WP. Benign ovarian cysts and ovarian cancer: A cohort study with implications for screening. *Lancet.* 2000;355:1060–3.

26. Alcázar JL, Martinez N, Juez L, Caparros M, Salas A, Errasti T. Ovarian simple cysts in asymptomatic postmenopausal women detected at transvaginal ultrasound: A review of literature. *World J Obstet Gynecol* 2015;4:108–12.

27. RCOG. *The management of ovarian cysts in postmenopausal women (Green-top Guideline No. 34).* July 2016.

28. Alcázar JL, Olartecoechea B, Guerriero S, Jurado M. Expectant management of adnexal masses in selected premenopausal women: A prospective observational study. *Ultrasound Obstet Gynecol.* 2013;41:582–8.

29. Suh-Burgmann E, Hung YY, Kinney W. Outcomes from ultrasound follow-up of small complex adnexal masses in women over 50. *Am J Obstet Gynecol.* 2014;211:623.e1–7.

30. Froyman W, Landolfo C, De Cock B, Wynants L, Sladkevicius P, Testa AC, Van Holsbeke C et al. Risk of complications in patients with conservatively managed ovarian tumours (IOTA5): A 2-year interim analysis of a multicentre, prospective, cohort study. *Lancet Oncol.* 2019;20:448–458.

31. Alcázar JL, Pascual MA, Marquez R, Ajossa S, Juez L, Graupera B, Piras A, Hereter L, Guerriero S. Malignancy risk of sonographically benign appearing purely solid adnexal masses in asymptomatic postmenopausal women. *Menopause.* 2017;24:613–6.

32. Caspi B, Appelman Z, Rabinerson D, Zalel Y, Tulandi T, Shoham Z. The growth pattern of ovarian dermoid cysts: A prospective study in premenopausal and postmenopausal women. *Fertil Steril.* 1997;68:501–5.

33. Hoo WL, Yazbek J, Holland T, Mavrelos D, Tong EN, Jurkovic D. Expectant management of ultrasonically diagnosed ovarian dermoid cysts: Is it possible to predict outcome? *Ultrasound Obstet Gynecol.* 2010;36:235–40.

34. Pascual MA, Graupera B, Pedrero C, Rodriguez I, Ajossa S, Guerriero S, Alcázar JL. Long-term results for expectant management of ultrasonographically diagnosed benign ovarian teratomas. *Obstet Gynecol.* 2017;130:1244–50.

35. Ssi-Yan-Kai G, Rivain AL, Trichot C, Morcelet MC, Prevot S, Deffieux X, De Laveaucoupet J. What every radiologist should know about adnexal torsion. *Emerg Radiol.* 2018;25:51–59.

36. Sasaki KJ, Miller CE. Adnexal torsion: Review of the literature. *J Minim Invasive Gynecol.* 2014;21:196–202.

37. Huchon C, Fauconnier A. Adnexal torsion: A literature review. *Eur J Obstet Gynecol Reprod Biol.* 2010;15:8–12.

38. Warner MA, Fleischer AC, Edell SL et al. Uterine adnexal torsion: Sonographic findings. *Radiology* 1985;154:773–5.

39. Kives S, Gascon S, Dubuc É, Van Eyk N. N° 341-Diagnostic et prise en charge de la torsion annexielle chez les filles, les adolescentes et les femmes adultes. *J Obstet Gynaecol Can.* 2017;39:91–100.

40. Chang HC, Bhatt S, Dogra VS. Pearls and pitfalls in diagnosis of ovarian torsion. *Radiographics.* 2008;28:1355–68.

41. Kiechl-Kohlendorfer U, Maurer K, Unsinn KM, Gassner I. Fluid-debris level in follicular cysts: A pathognomonic sign of ovarian torsion. *Pediatr Radiol.* 2006;36:421–5.

42. Sibal M. Follicular ring sign: A simple sonographic sign for early diagnosis of ovarian torsion. *J Ultrasound Med.* 2012;31:1803–9.

43. Albayram F, Hamper UM. Ovarian and adnexal torsion: Spectrum of sonographic findings with pathologic correlation. *J Ultrasound Med.* 2001;20:1083–9.

44. Bouguizane S, Bibi H, Farhat Y et al. Adnexal torsion: A report of 135 cases. *J Gynecol Obstet Biol Reprod* 2003;32:535–40.

45. Smorgick N, Maymon R, Mendelovic S, Herman A, Pansky M. Torsion of normal adnexa in postmenarcheal women: Can ultrasound indicate an ischemic process? *Ultrasound Obstet Gynecol.* 2008;31:338–41.

46. Shadinger LL, Andreotti RF, Kurian RL. Preoperative sonographic and clinical characteristics as predictors of ovarian torsion. *J Ultrasound Med.* 2008;27:7–13.

47. Lee EJ, Kwon HC, Joo HJ, Suh JH, Fleischer AC. Diagnosis of ovarian torsion with color Doppler sonography: Depiction of twisted vascular pedicle. *J Ultrasound Med.* 1998;17:83–9.

48. Vijayaraghavan SB. Sonographic whirlpool sign in ovarian torsion. *J Ultrasound Med.* 2004;23:1643–9.

49. Valsky DV, Esh-Broder E, Cohen SM, Lipschuetz M, Yagel S. Added value of the gray-scale whirlpool sign in the diagnosis of adnexal torsion. *Ultrasound Obstet Gynecol.* 2010;36:630–4.

50. Fleischer AC, Stein SM, Cullinan JA, Warner MA. Color Doppler sonography of adnexal torsion. *J Ultrasound Med.* 1995;14:523–8.

51. Tepper R, Zalel Y, Goldberger S, Cohen I, Markov S, Beyth Y. Diagnostic value of transvaginal color Doppler flow in ovarian torsion. *Eur J Obstet Gynecol Reprod Biol.* 1996;68:115–8.

52. Peña JE, Ufberg D, Cooney N, Denis AL. Usefulness of Doppler sonography in the diagnosis of ovarian torsion. *Fertil Steril.* 2000;73:1047–50.

CHAPTER 2

Pelvic Endometriosis

Stefano Guerriero, Silvia Ajossa, Alba Piras, Eleonora Musa, Virginia Zanda, Valerio Mais, and Anna Maria Paoletti

INTRODUCTION

Endometriosis is a chronic multifactorial disease. It is caused by the spread of endometrial glands and stroma outside the uterine cavity. Because of the subsequent growth of these ectopic implants, the woman affected presents with an inflammatory chronic process responsible for pelvic pain and severe dysfunction of the pelvic organs.[1]

The estimated prevalence in the general population is about 5%–10%.[2,3]

Endometriosis is a heterogeneous disease, so the patient can be completely asymptomatic or she can report dysmenorrhea, noncyclic chronic pelvic pain, dyspareunia, infertility, and urinary and intestinal disorders with a considerable negative impact on quality of life.[4] A close correlation with infertility and pelvic pain is reported, and in these women endometriosis is present in 25%–40% and 50% of the cases, respectively.[5,6] Another important factor correlated to this pathology is the presence of depressive and/or anxiety disorders and other kind of similar comorbidities that contribute to determine the high socioeconomic impact of this disease on health care expenses.[7,8]

Even if in most cases endometriosis causes several symptoms, a delay between the onset of symptomatology and diagnosis has been reported of 7–10 years.[8,9]

TRANSVAGINAL ULTRASOUND ASSESSMENT OF ENDOMETRIOSIS

The transvaginal ultrasound (TVS) is currently considered the first-line, noninvasive diagnostic method for the accurate diagnosis of deep infiltrative endometriosis (DIE) in rectosigmoid (RS) and in the other locations.[10-12]

There are three main types of endometriotic lesions: peritoneal (or superficial) endometriosis (SUP), ovarian endometrioma (OMA), and pelvic deep infiltrating endometriosis (DIE).

Ovarian Endometriosis

Currently, it is confirmed the high accuracy of TVS for the diagnosis of OMA, pelvic DIE, and pelvic adhesions associated with endometriosis, whereas SUP implants are not identifiable with TVS scans.[12]

The typical ultrasound (US) appearance of OMA (73%–82%[13] of OMAs) is a cystic lesion with "ground-glass" echogenicity (low-level homogeneous echogenic content corresponding to blood within the cystic cavity), well defined from the surrounding ovarian parenchyma, with no papillary projections or vascularized solid areas. This typical lesion is also known as a "chocolate cyst" (Figures 2.1 and 2.2). Less typical features include multiple locules (~85% with <5 locules), hyperechoic wall foci (Figure 2.3), cystic-solid lesion (~15%), solid lesion (1%), and anechoic cysts (rare, 2%).[12] The subjective impression of an expert US examiner is the main diagnostic method of OMAs with a positive predictive value of 86%, and also because of additional information achieved by the clinical history and pelvic exam.[12]

OMAs occur in about 17%–44% of women with endometriosis,[14] usually during the third and fourth decade of life. OMAs can be completely asymptomatic, or they can cause symptoms as pelvic pain, dysmenorrhea, and dyspareunia.[13] The left ovary is more frequently involved than the right one, and both are affected in 30%–50% of cases.[15]

The pathogenesis of OMA is still an object of debate. Many distinct theories have been proposed in literature, the most accredited ones being (1) the invagination of the ovarian cortex involved by active superficial ovarian implants, (2) the transformation of ovarian functional cyst in an endometriotic cyst, and (3) the "metaplastic potential of pelvic mesotelium."[16]

In literature, the risk of malignant transformation of an OMA has been reported as 0.6%–0.8% of the cases.[17]

In the US evaluation of a woman with a suspicion of ovarian OMA, it is important to consider that the US appearance of OMA differs between patients of distinct ages.

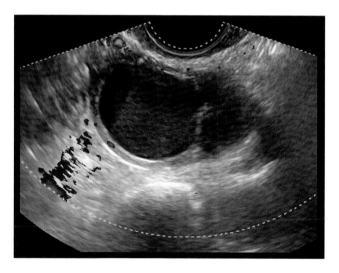

FIGURE 2.1 Transvaginal ultrasound showing the typical image of an endometrioma.

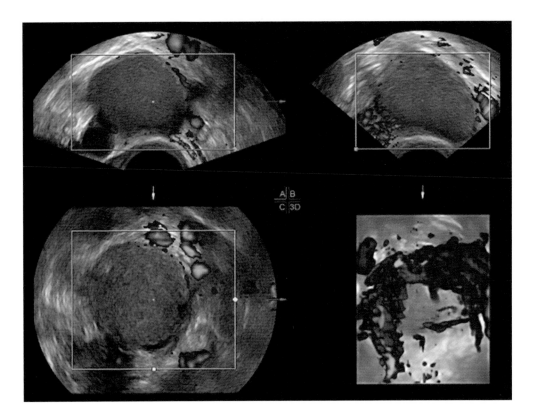

FIGURE 2.2   An endometrioma at three-dimensional color Doppler ultrasound.

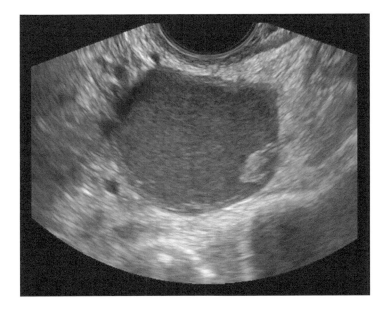

FIGURE 2.3   Endometrioma with hyperechoic wall foci.

The accurate and early diagnosis of OMA is important for several reasons:

- OMAs are considered to be *markers* for *posterior compartment* DIE, which is estimated to be found until in 98% of women with OMAs,[12] often associated with adhesions.

- A close relationship between OMAs and subfertility has been established.[18]

- OMAs may undergo decidualization in pregnancy, with problems of differential diagnosis with an ovarian malignancy,[19] even if the association with other endometriotic lesions may help in the diagnosis.[20]

- The diagnosis of OMAs at TVS can select the patients with an increased risk of complex pelvic disease, such as pelvic adhesions, pouch of Douglas (POD) obliteration, and endometriosis in the posterior compartment.

- OMA may also be associated with endometrioid adenocarcinoma and clear cell carcinoma of the ovary.[12,19]

Deep Infiltrating Endometriosis

A recent consensus statement on the systematic approach to sonographic evaluation of the pelvis in women with a clinical suspicion of endometriosis was published in 2016 by the International Deep Endometriosis Analysis (IDEA)[19] group with the contribution of clinicians, gynecological sonologists, advanced laparoscopic surgeons, and radiologists. The primary aim of IDEA consensus is to standardize terminology, definition of anatomy, measurements of sonographic features, and nomenclature of endometriosis lesions. The US examination in patients with suspected endometriosis has the goal to

1. Motivate the symptoms reported by the woman

2. Correctly map the endometriotic lesions to program the most appropriate treatment

3. Assess the severity of this pathology[19,21]

The systematic US approach proposed by the IDEA group includes four basic steps (Table 2.1).[19]

TABLE 2.1   Four Basic Sonographic Steps

First step	Routine evaluation of uterus and adnexa (plus sonographic signs of adenomyosis/presence or absence of endometrioma)
Second step	Evaluation of transvaginal sonographic "soft markers" (i.e., site-specific tenderness and ovarian mobility)
Third step	Assessment of status of POD using real-time ultrasound-based "sliding sign"
Fourth step	Assessment for DIE nodules in anterior and posterior compartments

Source: Guerriero S et al., *Ultrasound Obstet Gynecol.*, 2016;48:318–32. With permission.
Note: These steps can be adopted in this or any order as long as all four steps are performed to confirm/exclude the different forms of endometriosis.
Abbreviations: POD, pouch of Douglas.

First step: Using TVS, the operator should examine:

- The *uterus*, noting orientation (anteverted, retroverted, or axial), mobility (normal, reduced or fixed, "question mark sign"),[22] and any abnormalities. It is also important to evaluate the presence of signs of adenomyosis, and to describe them using the terms and definitions published in the Morphological Uterus Sonographic Assessment (MUSA)[23] consensus opinion.

- The *adnexa*, noting ovarian size and characteristics;[14] and the presence and number of OMAs, their measures on three orthogonal planes, and their US aspect,[24] using the International Ovarian Tumor Analysis (IOTA) terminology.[19,25] The US marker of "kissing ovaries" reflects the presence of severe pelvic adhesions.[19]

- The *fallopian tubes* (not usually visible on TVS if in a normal state) may appear distorted or fixed by adhesions in women with DIE. For this reason, it is important to consider endometriosis as a differential diagnosis in case of hydrosalpinx or hematosalpinx.[21]

Second step: The second step is a dynamic evaluation of *sonographic soft markers, site-specific tenderness* (SST), and *fixed ovaries*.[19] These "soft markers" are sonographic features that indirectly suggest the presence of endometriosis.[26,27] By applying pressure between the uterus and ovary, the US operator can evaluate if the ovary is fixed to the uterus, to the lateral pelvic side wall, or to the uterosacral ligaments (USLs). It is also possible to suspect the presence of adhesions palpating with the TVS probe and/or with the free hand on the abdominal wall.[19]

Third step: The third step is another dynamic real-time US technique to study the POD assessing the presence of a "sliding sign."

There are two distinct techniques depending on the orientation of the uterus. If the uterus is *anteverted* (Figure 2.4a), the operator can press gently with the TVS probe on

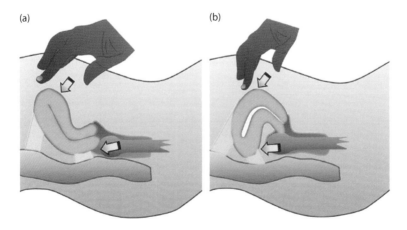

(a)　　　　　　　　　　　(b)

FIGURE 2.4　Schematic images demonstrating how to elicit the sliding sign in (a) an anteverted uterus and (b) a retroverted uterus. (From Guerriero S et al., *Ultrasound Obstet Gynecol.*, 2016;48:318–32. With permission.)

the cervix and evaluate if the anterior rectum glides freely (sliding sign is present) on the *posterior cervical and vaginal walls*. If the anterior rectal wall is fixed, the sliding sign is considered negative for the retrocervical region. Subsequently, the US operator puts one hand over the patient's lower anterior abdominal wall to try to move the uterus between the palpating hand and the TVS probe to evaluate if the anterior bowel glides freely (sliding sign is present) over the *posterior uterine wall*. When the sliding sign is assessed to be positive in the retrocervix region and in the posterior uterine wall, the POD is defined as "not obliterated."[19]

If the uterus is *retroverted* (Figure 2.4b), the US examiner gently presses with the TVS probe against the posterior upper uterine fundus to assess if the anterior rectal wall glides freely (sliding sign is present) across the posterior upper uterine fundus. The operator then puts one hand over the patient's lower anterior abdominal wall to try to move the uterus between the pushing hand and TVS probe, to evaluate if the anterior sigmoid glides freely (sliding sign is present) over the anterior lower uterine wall. When the sliding sign is assess to be positive in the posterior uterine fundus and the anterior lower uterine segment, the POD is defined "not obliterated."[19,28]

Fourth step: The fourth step consists in the US search of DIE nodules in the *anterior* and *posterior compartments* (Figure 2.5).[19]

The *anterior compartment* includes the urinary bladder, uterovesical pouch, and uterus. To evaluate this compartment, the operator can place the transducer in the anterior fornix of the vagina. In case of clinical suspicion of bladder endometriosis, the patient is advised to keep her bladder not completely empty (100–150 mL of urine).[19] The typical US aspect of endometriotic lesion of bladder is a hypoechoic linear or spherical lesion, with or without regular contours (Figures 2.6 and 2.7).[29–35] Using the sliding sign it is also possible to assess the presence of *uterovesical adhesions* that should be interpreted considering the patient's surgical history, such as previous cesarean sections.[21–36]

Endometriosis of the *posterior compartment* often involves the rectovaginal septum (RVS), POD/retrocervix, posterior vaginal wall/fornix, anterior rectum/rectosigmoid bowel, and pararectal space.[12] To evaluate this compartment, the operator can place the transducer in the posterior fornix of the vagina and slowly withdraw through the vagina.[19] *Lateral* pelvic DIE lesions can involve USLs, parametria, and the pelvic side wall.[12] The typical US appearances of DIE lesions within the posterior and lateral compartments are hypoechoic, not compressible and avascular.[12]

Rectovaginal septum (RSV): The rectovaginal area includes the vagina, the rectum, and the RVS. Furthermore, there is inconsistency in the definition of RV DIE in the literature.[19,37] Guerriero et al.[19] propose that involvement of the RVS should be suspected when a DIE nodule is seen on TVS in the rectovaginal space below the line passing along the lower border of the posterior lip of the cervix (under the peritoneum). Isolated RVS DIE is rare; RVS DIE (Figure 2.8) is usually considered an extension of the posterior vaginal wall, anterior rectal wall, or both posterior vaginal wall and anterior rectal wall involvement.[19,38] The use of TVS improves the detection of posterior vaginal and RVS DIE.[19,39,40]

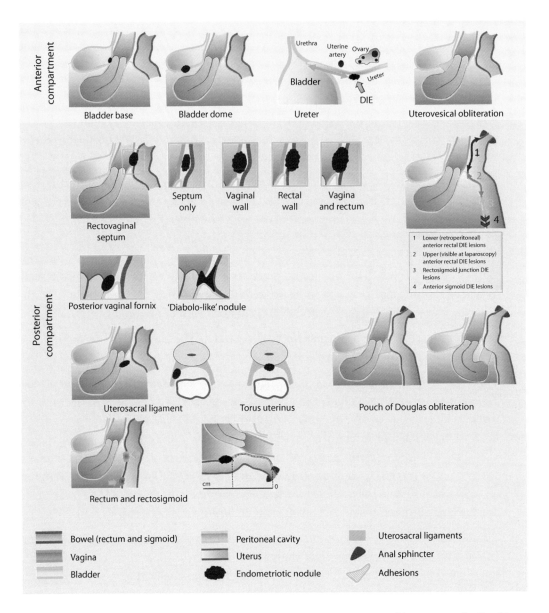

FIGURE 2.5 Schematic image of anterior and posterior compartmental locations of DIE. (From Guerriero S et al., *Ultrasound Obstet Gynecol.*, 2016;48:318–32. With permission.)

POD/retrocervix: The pouch of Douglas (POD) is a part of the female's peritoneum localized in the deepest region of pelvis between the lower posterior cervix and the anterior rectum. The term "complete obliteration of POD" refers to a situation in which this region is no longer visible because of adhesions, DE nodule, pelvic inflammatory disease (PID), or previous surgery.[41]

Posterior vaginal wall/fornix: This area is located at the vaginal vault, which is involved by DIE nodules mostly in the posterior vaginal fornix.[42] The typical US appearance of vaginal DIE nodules is an avascular lesion with an echogenicity similar to that of the normal vaginal

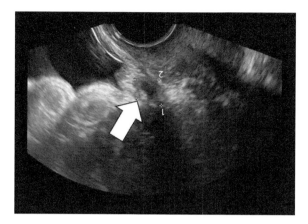

FIGURE 2.6   Transvaginal ultrasound depicting a bladder endometriotic nodule (arrow).

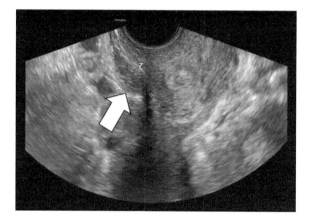

FIGURE 2.7   Transvaginal ultrasound depicting another bladder endometriotic nodule (arrow).

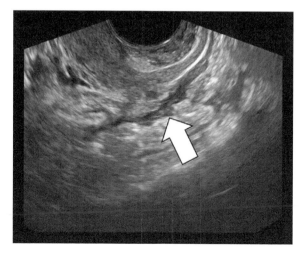

FIGURE 2.8   Transvaginal ultrasound depicting a rectovaginal endometriosis (arrow).

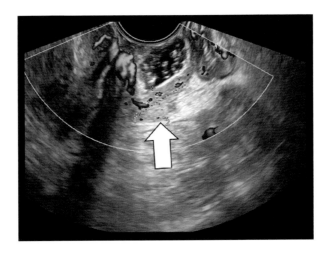

FIGURE 2.9   Transvaginal ultrasound depicting a forniceal endometriotic nodule (arrow).

mucosa.[12] A growing vaginal DIE nodule (Figures 2.9 through 2.11) often protrudes into the vaginal cavity, and it can be visualized by a speculum examination.

Rectum/rectosigmoid bowel: In this region DIE classically involves the anterior rectum, rectosigmoid junction, and/or sigmoid colon, all of which can be visualized using TVS. Bowel DIE can take the form of an isolated lesion or can be multifocal and/or multicentric. Bowel DIE usually appears on TVS as a thickening of the hypoechoic muscularis propria or as hypoechoic nodules, with or without hyperechoic foci with blurred margins (Figures 2.12 through 2.14).[19]

Uterosacral ligaments (USLs): Normal USLs are usually not visible on US. USL DIE lesions can be seen in the midsagittal view of the uterus. USLs are considered to be involved with DIE when a hypoechoic thickening with regular or irregular margins is seen within the peritoneal fat surrounding the USLs. This lesion may be isolated or part of a larger nodule extending into the vagina or into other surrounding structures. In some cases the

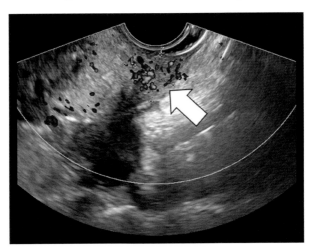

FIGURE 2.10   Transvaginal ultrasound depicting another forniceal endometriotic nodule (arrow).

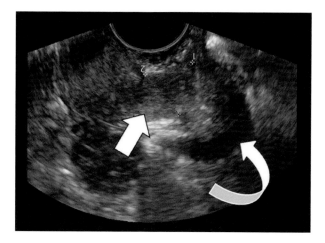

FIGURE 2.11   Transvaginal ultrasound depicting a nodule of fornix (straight arrow) associated with a rectosigmoid nodule (curved arrow).

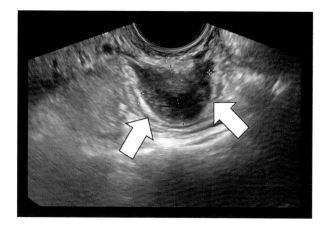

FIGURE 2.12   Transvaginal ultrasound depicting a rectosigmoid nodule (arrow).

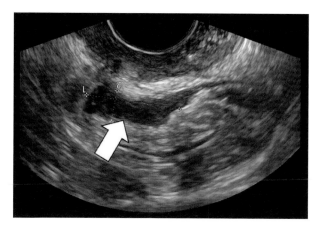

FIGURE 2.13   Transvaginal ultrasound depicting another rectosigmoid nodule (arrow).

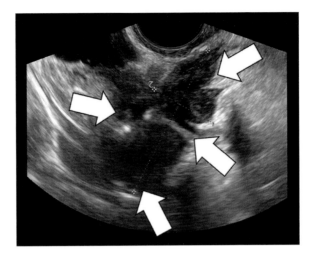

FIGURE 2.14   Transvaginal ultrasound depicting another huge rectosigmoid nodule (arrow).

DIE lesion involving the USL is located at the torus uterinus. If so, it is seen as a central thickening of the retrocervical area.[19] See Figures 2.15 and 2.16.

Several authors state that in expert hands this technique is a very accurate technique,[11,43–46] and a dedicated sonologist with specific knowledge is expected to have higher predictive accuracy.[47]

Unfortunately, some authors suggest that TVS for DIE is difficult to learn.[44] We totally disagree with this assumption. As a matter of fact, some found that after only one week of DIE TVS training, competency can be achieved within 40 procedures, enabling diagnosis of DIE with similar diagnostic accuracy as reported by centers of excellence.[48] Eisenberg et al.[49] also show that a sonographer trained in general gynecologic ultrasonography, who has invested time to learn TVS for DIE mapping, can achieve proficiency for diagnosing the major types of DIE lesions after examining fewer than 50 patients. In a recent study, we also observed that a 2-week learning program based on a mix of off-line and live sessions is feasible and suggests a good performance in training for the diagnosis of DIE.

As derived from some recent published meta-analyses, the overall diagnostic performance for DIE of the rectosigmoid is good with a sensitivity of 91% (95% CI: 85%–94%) and a

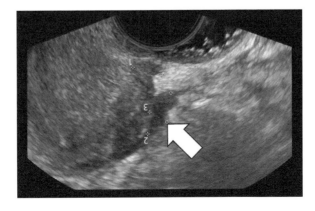

FIGURE 2.15   Transvaginal ultrasound depicting a uterosacral ligament nodule (arrow).

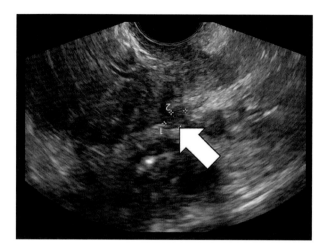

FIGURE 2.16   Transvaginal ultrasound depicting another uterosacral ligament nodule (arrow).

specificity of 97% (95% CI: 95%–98%),[45] while the overall diagnostic performance of TVS for detecting DIE in uterosacral ligaments, rectovaginal septum, vagina, and bladder is fair with high specificity.[11] In addition, the diagnostic performance of TVS and MRI is similar for detecting DIE involving the rectosigmoid, uterosacral ligaments, and rectovaginal septum.[46]

REFERENCES

1. Singh SS. "Endometriosis: Clinical and anatomical considerations." *How to Perform Ultrasonography in Endometriosis.* Guerriero S et al. (eds). Springer. 2018.
2. Vercellini P, Viganò P, Somigliana E, Fedele L. Endometriosis: Pathogenesis and treatment. *Nat Rev Endocrinol.* 2014;10(5):261–75.
3. Viganò P, Parazzini F, Somigliana E, Vercellini P. Endometriosis: Epidemiology and aetiological factors. *Best Pract Res Clin Obstet Gynaecol.* 2004;18(2):177–200.
4. Santulli P, Bourdon M, Presse M, Gayet V, Marcellin L, Prunet C, de Ziegler D, Chapron C. Endometriosis-related infertility: Assisted reproductive technology has no adverse impact on pain or quality-of-life scores. *Fertil Steril.* 2016;105:978–87.
5. Giudice LC. Clinical practice. *Endometriosis. N Engl J Med.* 2010;362:2389–98.
6. Somigliana E, Viganò P, Benaglia L, Busnelli A, Berlanda N, Vercellini P. Management of endometriosis in infertile patient. *Semin Reprod Med.* 2017;35(1):31–37.
7. Simoens S, Hummelshoj L, Dunselman G, Brandes I, Dirksen C, D'Hooghe T. Endometriosis cost assessment (the EndoCost study): A cost-of-illness study protocol. *Gynecol Obstet Invest.* 2011;71:170–6.
8. Hudelist G, Fritzer N, Thomas A, Niehues C, Oppelt P, Haas D, Tammaa A, Salzer H. Diagnostic delay for endometriosis in Austria and Germany: Causes and possible consequences. *Human Reproduction.* 2012;27(12):3412–6.
9. Matsuzaki S, Canis M, Pouly JL, Rabischong B, Botchorishvili R, Mage G. Relationship between delay of surgical diagnosis and severity of disease in patients with symptomatic deep infiltrating endometriosis. *Fertil Steril.* 2006;86:1314–6.
10. Exacoustos C, Manganaro L, Zupi E. Imaging for the evaluation of endometriosis and adenomyosis. *Best Pract Res Clin Obstet Gynaecol.* 2014;28:655–81.
11. Guerriero S, Ajossa S, Minguez JA, Jurado M, Mais V, Melis GB, Alcázar JL. Accuracy of transvaginal ultrasound for diagnosis of deep endometriosis in uterosacral ligaments,

rectovaginal septum, vagina and bladder: Systematic review and meta-analysis. *Ultrasound Obstet Gynecol.* 2015;46:534–545.

12. Reid S, Condous G. "Endometriomas and pelvic endometriosis." *Managing Ultrasonography in Human Reproduction: A Pratical Handbook.* Guerriero S et al. (eds). Springer. 2017.

13. Alcázar JL. "Ovarian endometriosis." *How to Perform Ultrasonography in Endometriosis.* Guerriero S et al. (eds). Springer. 2018.

14. Redwine DB. Ovarian endometriosis: A marker for more extensive pelvic and intestinal disease. *Fertil Steril.* 1999;72:310–5.

15. Al-Fozan H, Tulandi T. Left lateral predisposition of endometriosis and endometrioma. *Obstet Gynecol.* 2003;101:164–6.

16. Nisolle M, Donnez J. Peritoneal endometriosis, ovarian endometriosis, and adenomyotic nodules of the rectovaginal septum are three different entities. *Fertil Steril.* 1997;68:585–96.

17. Nishida M, Watanabe K, Sato N, Ichikawn Y. Malignant transformation of ovarian endometriosis. *Gynecol Obstet Investig.* 2000;50(Suppl 1):18–25.

18. Guerriero S, Van Calster B, Somigliana E et al. Age-related differences in the sonographic characteristics of endometriomas. *Hum Reprod.* 2016 August;31(8):1723–31.

19. Guerriero S, Condous G, Van der Bosch T et al. Systematic approach to sonographic evaluation of the pelvis in women with suspected endometriosis, including terms, definitions and measurements: A consensus opinion from the International Deep Endometriosis Analysis (IDEA) group. *Ultrasound Obstet Gynecol.* 2016;48:318–32.

20. Mascilini F, Moruzzi C, Giansiracusa C et al. Imaging in gynecological disease. 10: Clinical and ultrasound characteristics of decidualized endometriomas surgically removed during pregnancy. *Ultrasound Obstet Gynecol.* 2014;44:354–60.

21. Leonardi M, Condous G. "Standardized ultrasonographic diagnostic protocol to diagnose endometriosis based on the International Deep Endometriosis Analysis (IDEA) consensus statement." *How to Perform Ultrasonography in Endometriosis.* Guerriero S et al. (eds). Springer. 2018.

22. Di Donato N, Bertoldo V, Montanari G, Zannoni L, Caprara G, Seracchioli R. Question mark form of uterus: A simple sonographic sign associated with the presence of adenomyosis. *Ultrasound Obstet Gynecol.* 2015;46:126–7.

23. Van den Bosch T, Dueholm M et al. Terms, definitions and measurements to describe sonographic features of myometrium and uterine masses: A consensus opinion from the Morphological Uterus Sonographic Assessment (MUSA) group. *Ultrasound Obstet Gynecol.* 2015;46:284–98.

24. Van Holsbeke C, Van Calster B, Guerriero S et al. Endometriomas: Their ultrasound characteristics. *Ultrasound Obstet Gynecol.* 2010;35:730–40.

25. Timmerman D, Valentin L, Bourne TH, Collins WP, Verrelst H, Vergote I, International Ovarian Tumor Analysis Group. Terms, definitions and measurements to describe the sonographic features of adnexal tumors: A consensus opinion from the International Ovarian Tumor Analysis (IOTA) Group. *Ultrasound Obstet Gynecol.* 2000;16:500–5.

26. Redwine DB. Ovarian endometriosis: A marker for more extensive pelvic and intestinal disease. *Fertil Steril.* 1999;72:310–5.

27. Guerriero S, Ajossa S, Lai MP, Mais V, Paoletti AM, Melis GB. Transvaginal ultrasonography in the diagnosis of pelvic adhesions. *Hum Reprod.* 1997;12:2649–53.

28. Menakaya U, Condous G. The retroverted uterus: Refining the description of the real time dynamic "sliding sign." *Aust J Ultrasound Med.* 2013;16:97.

29. Hudelist G, Ballard K, English J et al. Transvaginal sonography vs clinical examination in the preoperative diagnosis of deep infiltrating endometriosis. *Ultrasound Obstet Gynecol.* 2011;37(4):480–7.

30. Fedele L, Bianchi S, Raffaelli R, Portuese A. Preoperative assessment of bladder endometriosis. *Hum Reprod.* 1997;12(11):2519–22.

31. Guerriero S, Ajossa S, Gerada M, Virgilio B, Angioni S, Melis GB. Diagostic value of transvaginal "tenderness-guided" ultrasonography for the prediction of deep endometriosis. *Hum Reprod.* 2008;23(11):2452–7.
32. Guerriero S, Ajossa S, Gerada M, D'Aquila M, Piras B, Melis GB. "Tenderness-guided" transvaginal ultrasonography: A new method for the detection of deep endometriosis in patients with chronic pelvic pain. *Fertil Steril.* 2007;88(5):1293–7.
33. Abrao MS, Goncalves MODC, Dias JA, Podgaec S, Chamie LP, Blasbalg R. Comparison between clinical examination, transvaginal sonography and magnetic resonance imaging for the diagnosis of deep endometriosis. *Hum Reprod.* 2007;22(12):3092–7.
34. Bazot M, Thomassin I, Hourani R, Cortez A, Darai E. Diagnostic accuracy of transvaginal sonography for deep pelvic endometriosis. *Ultrasound Obstet Gynecol.* 2004;24(2):180–5.
35. Savelli L, Manuzzi L, Pollastri P, Mabrouk M, Seracchioli R, Venturoli S. Diagnostic accuracy and potential limitations of transvaginal sonography for bladder endometriosis. *Ultrasound Obstet Gynecol.* 2009;34(5):595–600.
36. Moro F, Marvelos D, Pateman K, Holland T, Hoo WL, Jurkovic D. Prevalence of pelvic adhesions on ultrasound examination in women with a history of Cesarean section. *Ultrasound Obstet Gynecol.* 2015;45(2):223–8.
37. Reid S, Condous G. The issues surrounding the pre-operative TVS diagnosis of rectovaginal septum endometriosis. *Aust J Ultrasound Med.* 2014;17:2–3.
38. Reid S, Lu C, Hardy N, Casikar I, Reid G, Cario G, Chou D, Almashat D, Condous G. Office gel sonovaginography for the prediction of posterior deep infiltrating endometriosis: A multicenter prospective observational study. *Ultrasound Obstet Gynecol.* 2014;44:710–8.
39. Dessole S, Farina M, Rubattu G, Cosmi E, Ambrosini G, Nardelli GB. Sonovaginography is a new technique for assessing rectovaginal endometriosis. *Fertil Steril.* 2003;79:1023–7.
40. Saccardi C, Cosmi E, Borghero A, Tregnaghi A, Dessole S, Litta P. Comparison between transvaginal sonography, saline contrast sonovaginography and magnetic resonance imaging in the diagnosis of posterior deep infiltrating endometriosis. *Ultrasound Obstet Gynecol.* 2012;40:464–9.
41. Reid S. "Ultrasound in the evaluation of pouch of Douglas obliteration." *How to Perform Ultrasonography in Endometriosis.* Guerriero S et al. (eds). Springer. 2018.
42. Chapron C, Chopin N, Borghese B, Foulot H, Dousset B, Vacher-Lavenu MC, Viera M, Hasan W, Bricou A. Deeply infiltrating endometriosis: Pathogenetic implications of the anatomical distribution. *Hum Reprod.* 2006;21:1839–45.
43. Nisenblat V, Bossuyt PM, Farquhar C, Johnson N, Hull ML. Imaging modalities for the non-invasive diagnosis of endometriosis. *Cochrane Database Syst Rev.* 2016 February 26;2:CD009591.
44. Noventa M, Saccardi C, Litta P et al. Ultrasound techniques in the diagnosis of deep pelvic endometriosis: Algorithm based on a systematic review and meta-analysis. *Fertil Steril.* 2015;104:366–83.
45. Guerriero S, Ajossa S, Orozco R, Perniciano M, Jurado M, Melis GB, Alcázar JL. Accuracy of transvaginal ultrasound for diagnosis of deep endometriosis in the rectosigmoid: Systematic review and meta-analysis. *Ultrasound Obstet Gynecol.* 2016;47:281–9.
46. Guerriero S, Saba L, Pascual MA, Ajossa S, Rodriguez I, Mais V, Alcázar JL. Transvaginal ultrasound (TVS) versus magnetic resonance (MR) for diagnosing deep infiltrating endometriosis: A systematic review and meta-analysis. *Ultrasound Obstet Gynecol.* 2018;51:586–95.
47. Fraser MA, Agarwal S, Chen I, Singh SS. Routine vs. expert-guided transvaginal ultrasound in the diagnosis of endometriosis: A retrospective review. *Abdom Imaging.* 2015;40:587–94.
48. Piessens S, Healey M, Maher P, Tsaltas J, Rombauts L. Can anyone screen for deep infiltrating endometriosis with transvaginal ultrasound? *Aust N Z J Obstet Gynaecol.* 2014;54:462–8.
49. Eisenberg VH, Alcázar JL, Arbib N, Schiff E, Achiron R, Goldenberg M, Soriano D. Applying a statistical method in transvaginal ultrasound training: Lessons from the learning curve cumulative summation test (LC-CUSUM) for endometriosis mapping. *Gynecological Surgery.* 2017;14:19.

CHAPTER 3

Ovulation, Hemorrhagic Cyst, and Hyperstimulation Syndrome

María Ángela Pascual and Jean L. Browne

INTRODUCTION

The ovary has a complex structure, composed of various different tissues (Figure 3.1), including epithelial cells, germinal cells (intrafollicular oocytes), fibroconnective tissue, and follicular cells (in the theca and the granulosa). Therefore, from each individual tissue may arise a wide variety of benign and malign tumors.

During the follicular phase, numerous follicles start developing. One of them will become the dominant follicle, then progress to the preovulatory stage or De Graaf follicle.

Ovulation and yellow body formation happen near the 14th day in a 28-day cycle. It starts with the De Graaf follicle rupturing and freeing the oocyte and follicular liquid in the peritoneal cavity. Granulosa cells are infiltrated by new blood vessels, and the internal theca and granulosa cells develop lipidic granulations and a yellow pigment, giving rise to the yellow body or corpus luteum. If there is no fecundation, the yellow body will last about 14 days and then give way to a fibrous scar called corpus albicans (Figure 3.2a–e).

Alterations to this physiologic cycle can happen at any stage. Dysfunctional cycles are mostly seen during adolescence and during perimenopause, that is to say at the beginning or the end of the women's fertility stage. These dysfunctions are frequent, and can have acute and very intense symptomatology that is self-limited but might induce unrequired surgical procedures. Hospitalization for this reason happens in about 500/100,000.[1] Prevalence of these dysfunctional findings vary according to the cohort being studied, with ranges from 14% to 66% (Table 3.1).

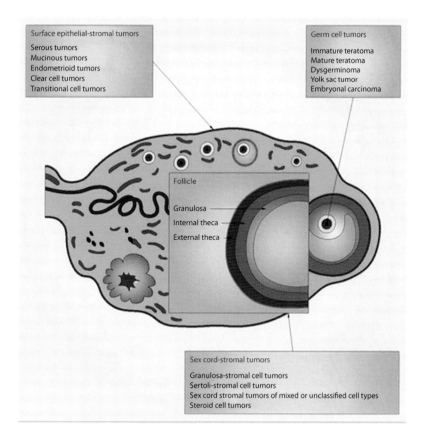

FIGURE 3.1   Drawing showing the wide variety of cell types of the ovary.

Ultrasonographic diagnosis of the functional findings of the ovary is done using IOTA terminology regarding size, ultrasonographic structural characteristics, and vascularization.[2] Morphologic ultrasound findings are just one of the main diagnostic pillars and have to be correlated with anamnesis, namely, hormonal state, clinical examination, and chemistry, including tumor markers.

In our experience, 85% of ultrasound findings of dysfunctional origin spontaneously unravel.[3] In a study by Alcázar et al., functional cysts regressed in 84% of cases. Other authors have reported spontaneous resolution of dysfunctional ovarian findings in 75%[5] and in 89% of cases.[6] These include different disruptions of normal evolution of the ovarian cycle, such as follicular persistence (Figure 3.3), luteinized follicle without follicle rupture or LUF (luteinized unruptured follicle) (Figure 3.4) when no ovulation has occurred, and, if ovulation has happened, alterations in the corpus luteum, which can lead to hemorrhagic cysts (Figure 3.5).

FOLLICLE PERSISTENCE

Follicle persistence happens when the follicle does not rupture and continues growing past 30 mm. Diagnosis requires serial ultrasound examinations and hormonal measurements. The cystic follicle is anechoic, with clearly defined borders and no

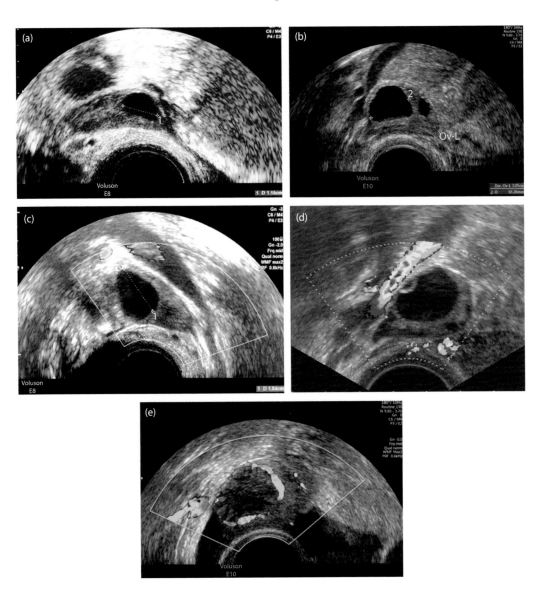

FIGURE 3.2 (a) Sonogram of ovary with a dominant follicle at the beginning of the follicular phase. (b) The follicle grows 1–2 mm per day. (c) Image showing an 18 mm follicle. (d) Transvaginal sonogram of the ovary containing a preovulatory follicle with a cumulus oophorus during the moment of presumed ovulation. (e) Transvaginal color Doppler scan of the ovary. Increased vascularity of the corpus luteum is easily seen by color flow imaging, the "ring of fire."

TABLE 3.1   Prevalence of Functional Cysts Reported in Different Series

Author	%
M. Vessey[17]	66.0
R. Osmers[6]	53.0
J.L. Alcázar[4]	36.5
M.A. Pascual[3]	14.0

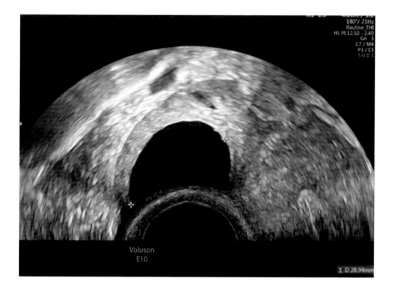

FIGURE 3.3 Transvaginal ultrasound showing right ovary, with an anechoic image of regular contours and without internal echoes of almost 30 mm, illustrating the typical image of a follicular persistence.

septa or internal diffuse echoes or proliferations. The endometrium is thickened and hyperechoic (Figure 3.6).

During its evolution, intrafollicular bleeding may occur in a persistent follicle, and the sonographic pattern becomes more complex, with diffuse echoes and gravitational deposits, or septa may become evident, resembling a hemorrhagic corpus luteum.

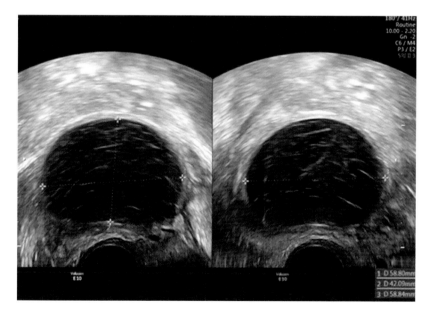

FIGURE 3.4 Transvaginal sonogram shows a luteinized unruptured follicle (LUF). Note thin septa within the cyst cavity.

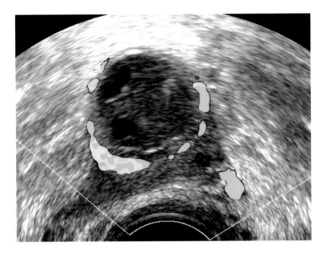

FIGURE 3.5 Color Doppler image of corpus luteum with hemorrhagic phenomena. Note the peripheral vascularization.

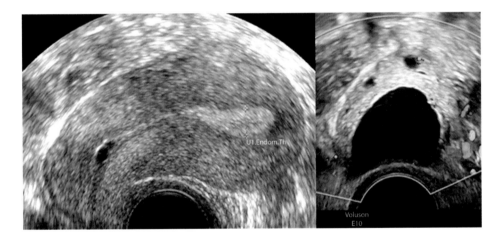

FIGURE 3.6 Image showing follicular persistence in the right ovary. Note in the left image transversal scan of a secretory endometrium.

The plain anechoic pattern in a large cyst is not exclusive to a persistent follicle. Differential diagnosis includes serous cystadenoma or even a mucinous cyst without septa. Diagnosis is certain when spontaneous involution of a persistent follicle happens after menses, although sometimes complete disappearance can take two or three menstrual cycles.

LUTEINIZED UNRUPTURED FOLLICLE OR LUF

An LUF occurs when the follicle doesn't rupture but the luteal phase takes place.[7] LUFs generally involute spontaneously, also spanning one to three cycles. Its sonographic pattern is more complex than a follicular cyst. They may grow considerably, reaching 80–100 mm in diameter (Figure 3.7). Signs of luteinization are thickening of the cyst's wall, diffuse echoes, and especially evidence of fine septa.

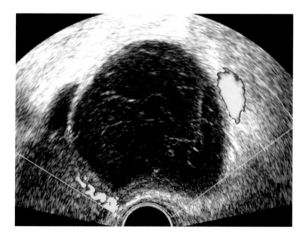

FIGURE 3.7   Image showing a unilocular cyst of regular contour and thin septa inside, characteristic features of luteinized unruptured follicles (LUFs).

As with a persistent follicle, an LUF's spontaneous involution is diagnostic. Differential diagnosis is mainly with an endometriosis cyst due to the presence of diffuse intracystic echoes.[8]

Women on low-dose monophasic oral contraceptive treatment have a lower prevalence of functional cysts than those who do not, with a relative risk of developing functional ovarian cyst of 0.22 (95% CI: 0.13–0.39).[9]

FUNCTIONAL HEMORRHAGIC CYSTS

Both an LUF and a persistent cyst may give rise to a hemorrhagic cyst, but the normal rupture of the follicle during ovulation is also a traumatic event that produces bleeding, engendering a hemorrhagic corpus luteum with hemoperitoneum (Figure 3.8), therefore with acute and intense pelvic pain.[10]

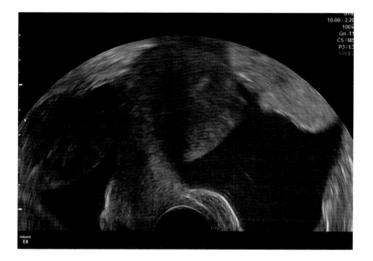

FIGURE 3.8   Sonographic findings reveal free fluid, frequently with diffuse echoes (hemoperitoneum) after rupture of a functional hemorrhagic cyst.

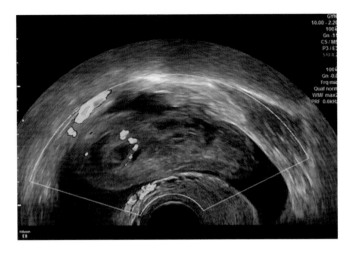

FIGURE 3.9 Sonogram of spontaneous resolution of a hemorrhagic LUF with a heterogeneous, apparently solid pattern.

Sonographic findings reveal free fluid in the Douglas pouch, frequently with diffuse echoes (as befits hemoperitoneum). These cysts are heterogeneous and may vary their morphology within days. Their borders may be hard to distinguish and irregular (Figure 3.9), they may have septa, and even present apparent solid proliferations that really are vascularized blood clots (Figure 3.10), even requiring differential diagnosis with a malignant cyst due to the complex pattern and physiologic angiogenesis of the corpus luteum. Other causes of acute pelvic pain include ectopic pregnancy and appendicitis. Serum β-HCG can help diagnose a hemorrhagic cyst. As per IOTA descriptions[2] of hemorrhagic cysts, the pattern may be star-shaped (Figure 3.11), cobweb-like, or jelly-like (Figure 3.12).[11]

Jain et al.[12] described the hemorrhagic cyst, stressing the good sonographic transmission through the cyst due to its mainly liquid nature.

Most of these functional entities are usually unilateral, are seen without ovulation induction treatment, and disappear spontaneously in a three menstrual cycle span.

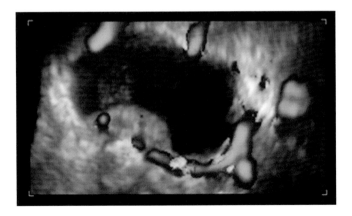

FIGURE 3.10 Image showing a three-dimensional ultrasound of a hemorrhagic corpus luteum, with an apparent solid proliferation.

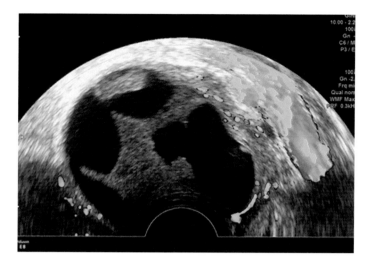

FIGURE 3.11   Sonogram showing a hemorrhagic cyst that may occasionally seem partially solid, due to dense internal echoes. This may be seen in the subacute stage, when there is blood clot formation and the clot lysis has not yet begun. Notice the internal star-shaped pattern.

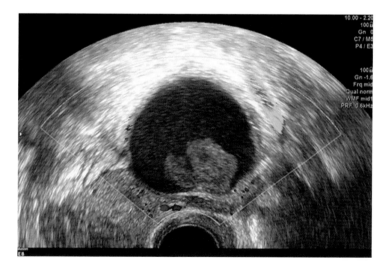

FIGURE 3.12   Transvaginal scan of hemorrhagic cyst. Note the echogenic content due to a clot within the blood-filled cystic cavity. This is the jelly-like pattern.

With respect to the management of hemorrhagic cysts, the Society of Radiologists in Ultrasound Consensus Conference Statement indicates the following:[13]

- Premenopausal women

  - No ultrasound follow-up needed unless there's an uncertain diagnosis or if the cyst is larger than 5 cm

  - More than 5 cm cyst diameter: Follow-up ultrasound in 6–12 weeks

- Recently menopausal women

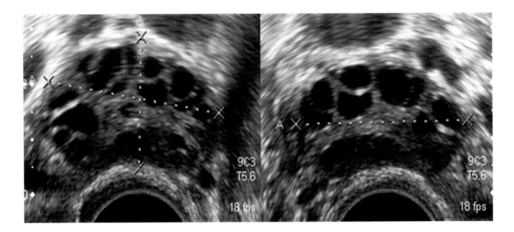

FIGURE 3.13 Transvaginal ultrasound showing a polycystic ovary (PCO) with more than 20 follicles with diameters between 2–9 mm.

- Ultrasound follow-up in 6–12 weeks to confirm resolution of the initial findings
- Late menopausal women
  - Possible non-benign cyst; considere surgical removal

OVARIAN HYPERSTIMULATION

The ovarian hyperstimulation syndrome (OHS) may occur in women receiving gonadotropins, or less frequently clomiphene citrate, to induce ovulation during assisted reproduction treatment. This exaggerated ovarian response may give rise to serious complications

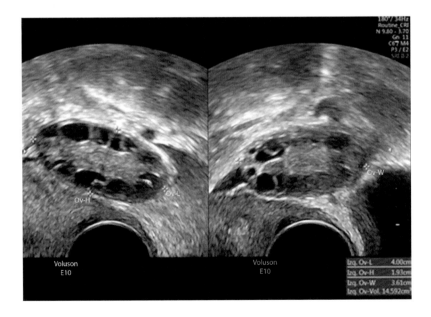

FIGURE 3.14 Sonogram of the polycystic ovary. A large number of small cystic structures are crowded together and stand out in the enlarged ovarian stroma (14.59 cc).

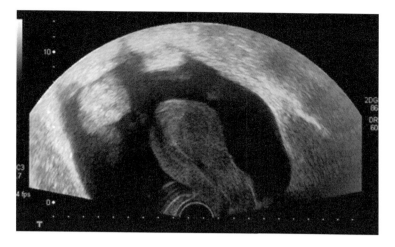

FIGURE 3.15   Sonogram showing a large amount of fluid in the pouch of Douglas.

such as thromboembolic phenomena, kidney failure, liver dysfunction, or bleeding due to a ruptured ovary. An endogenous rise of gonadotropins is also rarely a cause of OHS.

The physiologic pathway to OHS is borne through an elevated capillary permeability leading to the creation of a large amount of extravascular fluid, diminished intravascular volume, and organ perfusion, which are reflected in its main symptoms (i.e., ascites, hypotension and oliguria).

One risk factor associated with OHS developing in women treated to induce ovulation is a polycystic ovary (PCO) (Figure 3.13). One ovary with more than 20 follicles with diameters between 2 and 9 mm and/or an ovarian volume >10 cc is considered a PCO (Figure 3.14).[14]

Suspicion of OHS is warranted by ultrasound findings of an enlarged ovary, fluid in the pouch of Douglas (Figure 3.15) and abdominal ascites (Figure 3.16).[15]

According to the ovary's size, less than 6 cm is mild OHS (Figure 3.17), moderate from 6 to 12 cm (Figure 3.18), and severe if the ovarian size exceeds 12 cm (Figure 3.19).[16]

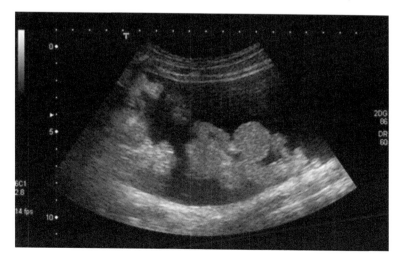

FIGURE 3.16   Image showing abdominal ascites in a severely hyperstimulated patient.

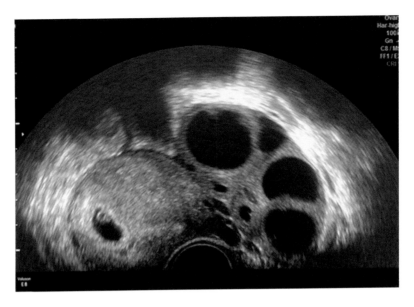

FIGURE 3.17 Transvaginal ultrasound showing an incipient pregnancy, with a mildly hyperstimulated ovary.

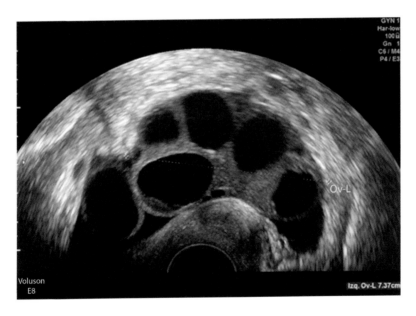

FIGURE 3.18 Image showing a moderately hyperstimulated ovary.

ACKNOWLEDGMENTS

Under the auspices of the Càtedra d' Investigació en Obstetrícia i Ginecologia de la Universitat Autònoma de Barcelona. Thanks to Beatriz Valero for help in the editing of this work.

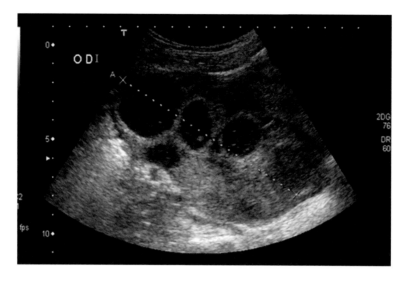

FIGURE 3.19   Sonogram showing a severely hyperstimulated ovary (more than 120 mm).

REFERENCES

1. Grimes DA, Hugues JM. Use of multiphasic oral contraceptives and hospitalizations of women with functional ovarian cysts in the United States. *Obstet Gynecol.* 1989;73:1037–9.
2. Timmerman D, Valentin L, Bourne TH, Collins WP, Verrelst H, Vergote I. Terms, definitions and measurements to describe the sonographic features of adnexal tumors: A consensus opinion from the International Ovarian Tumor Analysis (IOTA) Group. *Ultrasound Obstet Gynecol.* 2000;16:500–5.
3. Pascual MA, Hereter L, Tresserra F, Carreras O, Ubeda A, Dexeus S. Transvaginal sonographic appearance of functional ovarian cysts. *Hum Reprod.* 1997;12:1246–49.
4. Alcázar JL, Errasti T, Jurado M. Blood flow in functional cysts and benign ovarian neoplasms in premenopausal women. *J Ultrasound Med.* 1997;16:819–24.
5. Fleischer AC, Cullinan JA, Jones HW, Peery CV, Bluth RF, Kepple DM. Serial assessment of adnexal masses with transvaginal color Doppler sonography. *Ultrasound Med Biol.* 1995;21:435–41.
6. Osmers RG, Osmers M, Von Maydell B, Wagner B, Kuhn W. Preoperative evaluation of ovarian tumors in the premenopause by transvaginosonography. *Am J Obstet Gynecol.* 1996;175:428–34.
7. Hamilton CJ, Wetzels LC, Evers JL, Hoggland HJ, Muitjens A, de Haan J. Follicle growth curves and hormonal patterns in patients with the luteinized unruptured follicle syndrome. *Fert Steril.* 1985;43:541–8.
8. Pascual MA, Tresserra F, Lopez-Marin L, Ubeda A, Grase PJ, Dexeus S. Role color Doppler ultrasonography in the diagnosis of endometriotic cysts. *JUM* 2000;19:695–9.
9. Christensen JT, Boldsen JL, Westergaard JG. Functional ovarian cysts in premenopausal and gynecologically healthy women. *Contraception* 2002;66:153–7.
10. Abbas AM, Amin MT, Tolba SM, Ali MK. Hemorrhagic ovarian cysts: Clinical and sonographic correlation with the management options. *Middle East Fertility Soc J.* 2016;21:41–5.
11. Guerriero S, Ajossa S, Gerada M et al. Transvaginal ultrasonography in the diagnosis of extrauterine pelvic disease. *Exp Rev Obstet Gynecol.* 2008;3:731–52.
12. Jain KA. Sonographic spectrum of hemorrhagic ovarian cysts. *J Ultrasound Med.* 2002;21:879–86.

13. Levine D, Brown DL, Andreotti RF et al. Management of asymptomatic ovarian and other adnexal cysts imaged at US: Society of Radiologists in Ultrasound Consensus Conference Statement. *Radiology* 2010;256:943–54.
14. The International PCOS Network. *International evidence-based guideline for the assessment and management of polycystic ovary syndrome.* Melbourne, Australia. Monash University. 2018.
15. Humaidan P, Quartarolo J, Evangelos G, Papanikolaou EG. Preventing ovarian hyperstimulation syndrome: Guidance for the clinician. *Fertil Steril.* 2010;94:389–400.
16. Gola A, Ron-el R, Herman A, Soffer Y, Weinraub Z, Caspi E. Ovarian hyperstimulation syndrome: An update review. *Obstet Gyanecol Surv.* 1989;44:430–40.
17. Vessey M, Metcalfe A, Wells C, McPherson K, Westhoff C, Yeates D. Ovarian neoplasms, functional ovarian cysts, and oral contraceptives. *Br Med J.* 1987;294:1518–20.

CHAPTER 4

Pelvic Inflammatory Disease

Stefano Guerriero, Silvia Ajossa, Alba Piras, Eleonora Musa, Virginia Zanda, Valerio Mais, and Anna Maria Paoletti

INTRODUCTION

Pelvic inflammatory disease (PID) is a pathology of a woman's reproductive organs that originates from an infectious process spread through the cervix to the uterus, fallopian tubes up to the ovaries, and pelvic peritoneum.[1]

Frequently, this disease is not correctly diagnosed because of high rates of subclinical cases of this disease, and, for this reason, the real incidence is underestimated.[2] The prevalence has been valuated in 9–27/1000 women in reproductive age.[3,4]

PID is caused by bacteria, most of which are sexually transmitted, such as *Chlamydia trachomatis* and *Neisseria gonorrhoeae*. The transmission may occur during unprotected sexual intercourse, but also in the case of childbirth, miscarriage, or use of spiral contraception.

This pathology is part of the "nonspecific lower abdominal pain syndrome" (NSLAP) in women in reproductive age, and its clinical presentation is variable and in close correlation with the anatomical relationship between the reproductive organs, the menstrual cycle, and pregnancy.[5]

PID is the main gynecological cause of acute pelvic pain in the women,[6] but in many cases it is completely asymptomatic. The most frequent symptoms are lower abdominal pain, fever, symptoms of lower genital tract infection (abnormal vaginal discharge or bleeding, itching and odor, difficult or pain in urination), and dyspareunia. It is important to consider the possible severe short- and long-term sequelae of a PID not readily diagnosed and treated, such as infertility and ectopic pregnancy (for damage of the fallopian tubes), and pelvic chronic pain, which contribute to the increase of associated psycho-physical stress.[1]

The sensitivity of the clinical diagnosis of PID is of 60%–70%.[7] Actually, the main diagnostic method is laparoscopy, but it has not demonstrated its reproducibility for the diagnosis of this patology,[8] and moreover, it exposes the patient to a risk of complications, and it is expensive and invasive.[9]

ULTRASOUND FINDINGS IN PELVIC INFLAMMATORY DISEASE

Several studies in the past years[10–20] showed that tubal inflammatory disease presents the following transvaginal ultrasonographic features ("soft markers") that are typical and reproducible for ultrasound (US) expert examiners:[21]

  I. Shape: A pear elongated-shaped structure with anechoic or low-level content.

  II. Wall with

    a. Incomplete septa, which appear as hyperechoic septa, that originate from one side of the wall, but do not arrive to the opposite side (Figure 4.1).

    b. "Cogwheel sign,"[19] which appears in the cross section (Figure 4.2).

    c. "Waist sign," defined as diametrically opposed indentations along the wall of the cystic mass (Figure 4.3) described by Patel et al.[20]

    d. "Beads-on-a-string" sign, defined as hyperechoic wall nodules of 2–3 mm (Figure 4.4).

  III. Wall thickness is defined as thick if ≥5 mm and thin if it <5 mm.

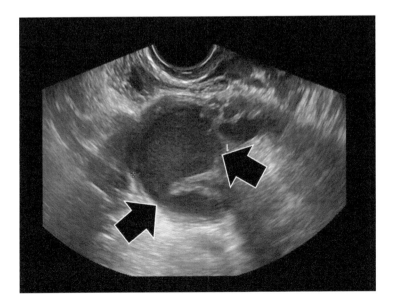

FIGURE 4.1 Transvaginal ultrasound showing an incomplete septa in a case of acute tubal inflammatory disease with a tube filled with hypoechoic fluid.

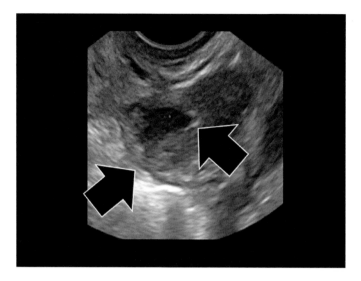

FIGURE 4.2 Transvaginal ultrasound showing the cogwheel sign (arrows) in a case of acute tubal inflammatory disease.

IV. Extension to the ovaries

    a. Absent, if the ovaries are normal.

    b. Tubo-ovarian complex (TOC), defined by the well identification of the ovary and the tube, which cannot be separated by pushing with the vaginal US probe in a woman with symptoms of acute pelvic inflammatory disease (Figure 4.5). This lesion can be unilateral or bilateral.

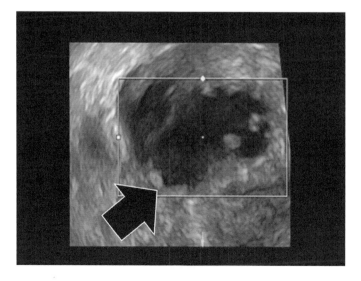

FIGURE 4.3 Transvaginal ultrasound showing the waist sign (defined as diametrically opposed indentations along the wall of the cystic mass). (As described by Patel MD et al. *AJR Am J Roentgenol*, 2006 April;186:1033–8.)

    c. Tubo-ovarian abscess (TOA), defined by the presence of a painful mass in which the ovary and the tube are not easily identified, and it is not possible to separate them by pushing with the vaginal US probe. This lesion can be unilateral or bilateral, associated or not with the presence of corpuscolated fluid in the pouch of Douglas.

V. Free fluid or a peritoneal inclusion cyst, defined by the presence of an anechoic "fluid-filled accumulation in the cul-de-sac" whose walls are constituted by the peritoneum, without tenderness by pushing with the probe.[21,22]

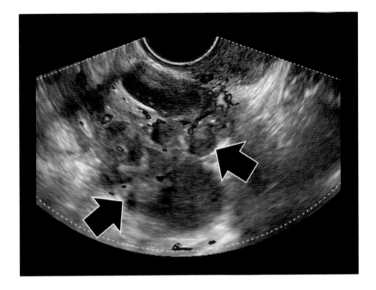

FIGURE 4.4 Transvaginal ultrasound showing the presence of beads-on-a-string signs (small hyperechoic mural nodules; arrows).

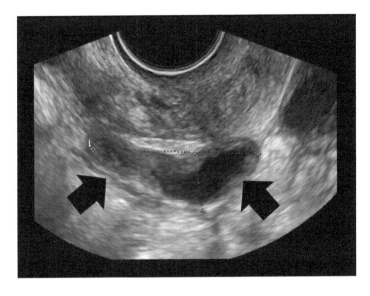

FIGURE 4.5 Transvaginal ultrasound showing a tubo-ovarian complex (TOC).

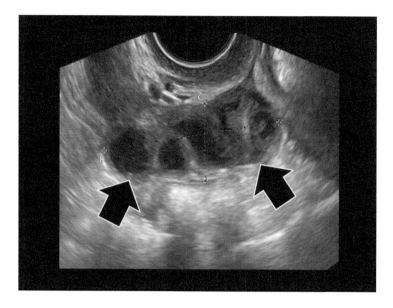

FIGURE 4.6   Transvaginal ultrasound showing a thick fallopian tube wall in a case of acute tubal inflammatory disease.

The natural history of this pathology starts from an initial acute inflammatory phase of the tubal wall, which appears thick (Figures 4.6 and 4.7) and edematous (cogwheel sign), with mucinous or purulent tubal content that can arrive externally in the pelvic cavity.[10,21]

In case of the lumen's occlusion in the distal portion of the tube, the mucinous or purulent content extends the tubal walls inducing hydrosalpinx or pyosalpinx. Then,

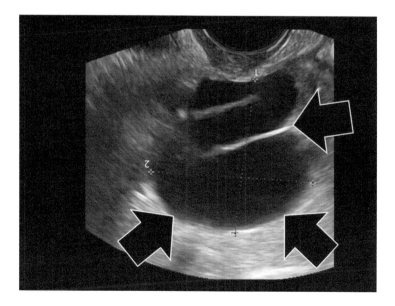

FIGURE 4.7   Transvaginal ultrasound showing another thick fallopian tube wall in a case of acute tubal inflammatory disease.

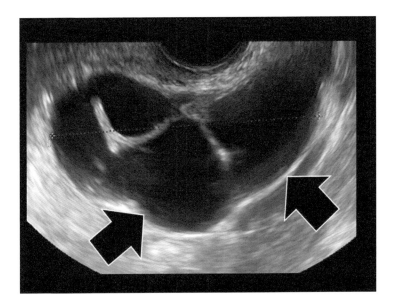

FIGURE 4.8   Transvaginal ultrasound showing incomplete septa in case of hydrosalpinx.

the tube appears on US as retort-shaped tubes with the presence of incomplete septa and beads-on-a-string sign, both in the acute and chronic phase (Figures 4.8 and 4.9).[22] If the tubal patency persists, one or more microbial agents can reach the ovary. Especially if this occurs during the ovulation, the bacteria can penetrate inside the ovary with the subsequent spread of the inflammatory process and formation of the TOC, that on US imaging show inflammatory features, such as a thick tubal wall or cogwheel sign. At this

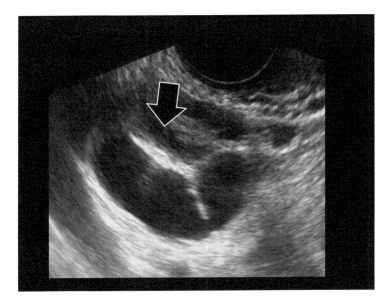

FIGURE 4.9   Transvaginal ultrasound showing other incomplete septa in case of hydrosalpinx.

time, the medical/surgical treatment can generally restore the normal anatomy, but if this stage is exceeded, in the following days the process can evolve toward the formation of an abscess (TOA) with a complete breakdown of the adnexal features, and can extend the inflammation to the contralateral adnexa, in which starts the formation of a TOC.[22]

In the chronic phase, which occurs if a medical or surgical treatment is not applied and there is not a spontaneous resolution of the process, the presence of fluid persists into the conglomerate tube[21] and tubal walls are thin, less than 5 mm (Figure 4.10).

Several authors[12-23] use TOC and TOA incorrectly as synonyms. We have previously explained that these two definitions refer to two different phases of the same disease, which appear at the ultrasound exam differently and benefit from distinct treatments.[22]

A sensitivity of 93% and a specificity of 98% for the ultrasonographic diagnosis of TOA is reported,[24] and this accuracy can improve with the use of power Doppler (PD) technique, detecting the typical hyperemia associated to the inflammatory process.[25,26]

Molander et al.[8] showed the possibility to correctly distinguish between acute PID (often with tubal patency) and nonacute hydrosalpinx (with a pyosalpinx formation) using the transvaginal ultrasound technique (TVS).[27,28] Moreover, they focused their attention on the tubal wall thickness, recommending that a thickness >5 mm associated with the US marker of cogwheel sign are strongly indicative of acute PID; while, the US marker of incomplete septa (Figures 4.11 and 4.12) can be detectable in acute PID and nonacute hydrosalpinx (Figures 4.13 through 4.15). A new important US marker is the finding at PD of *multiple blood vessels in the thickened wall* during the acute PID (Figure 4.16), with lower flow impedance (FI) than in hydrosalpinx, whilst the pulsatility index (PI) are comparable in these two (acute PID and hydrosalpinx).[9,22]

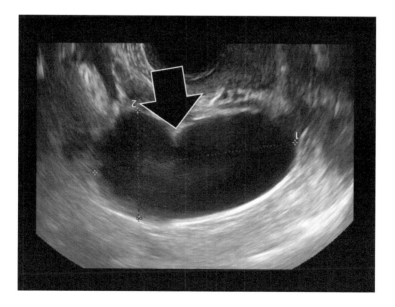

FIGURE 4.10 Transvaginal ultrasound showing a thin fallopian tube wall (less than 5 mm) in a case of chronic tubal inflammatory disease surrounding the ovary.

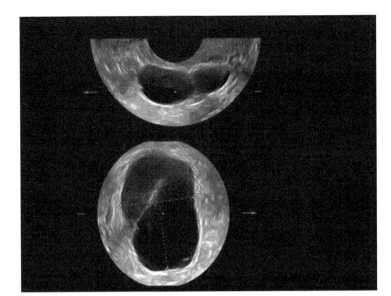

FIGURE 4.11 Three-dimensional ultrasound showing 3D rendering of the coronal plane, improving the visualization of incomplete septa.

It's important to make a correct differential diagnosis between PID and rupture of active endometrioma, which causes an important pelvic inflammatory process highly vascularized at PD detection in a patient with acute pelvic pain.[29]

Regarding the US features of PID with the use of color Doppler TVS, Kupesic et al.[30] reported that 76% of women with acute PID showed an adnexal mass vascularized at color

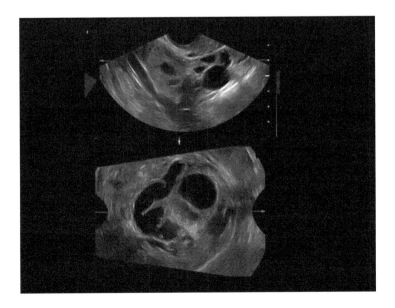

FIGURE 4.12 Another 3D rendering of the coronal performed to improve the visualization of incomplete septa.

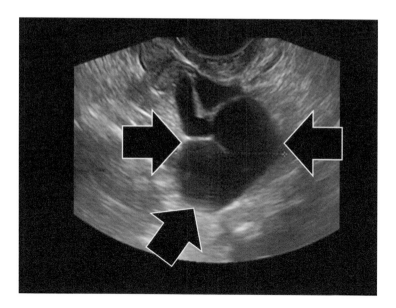

FIGURE 4.13   In this case, the hydrosalpinx appears as multilocular, but by rotating the probe the incomplete septum is visualized in the majority of cases.

Doppler evaluation with a resistance blood flow index (RI) to be lower in acute PID than the chronic phase (Figure 4.17),[30] which was also subsequently confirmed by Alatas et al.[31]

Other authors[32] reported that RI of the fallopian tube's artery decreases directly proportionally with severity of the acute pelvic inflammatory process, because of the hyperemia associated, while the same vascular index increases in case of resolution of

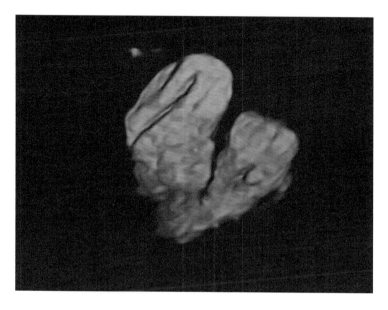

FIGURE 4.14   Three-dimensional ultrasound showing 3D inversion rendering mode of a hydrosalpinx.

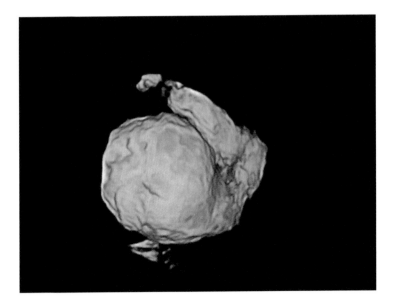

FIGURE 4.15   Three-dimensional ultrasound showing another 3D inversion-rendering mode of a hydrosalpinx.

the inflammatory phase. However, the PD technique provides more information in the evaluation of PID than the conventional color Doppler, such as the capacity to show areas of undetectable flow.[33] However, high US experience is fundamental, because the PD technique also has some limits, such as the creation of motion artifacts (often due to bowel movements) and flashes from pelvic vessels close to the adnexa. Thus, the TVS

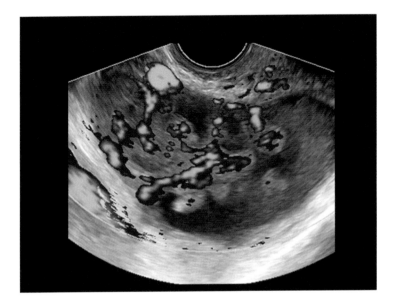

FIGURE 4.16   Transvaginal color Doppler ultrasound depicting intense vascularization (color score 4) in a case of acute tubal inflammatory disease.

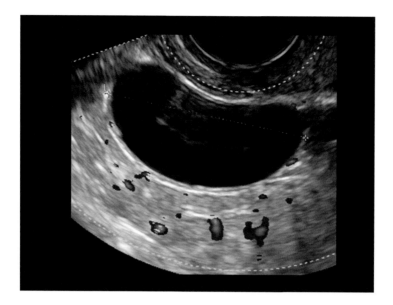

FIGURE 4.17 Transvaginal color Doppler ultrasound depicting few vascular spots (color score 2) in case of a chronic tubal inflammatory disease.

method performed by US expert examiners associated with the power Doppler technique can be considered the first choice diagnostic method to diagnose PID, as it is accurate, reproducible,[9] and noninvasive.

REFERENCES

1. Crossman SH. The challenge of pelvic inflammatory disease. *Am Fam Physician.* 2006;73:859–64.
2. Lareau SM, Beigi RH. Pelvic inflammatory disease and tubo-ovarian abscess. *Infect Dis Clin N Am.* 2008;22:693–708.
3. Gogate A, Brabin L, Nicholas S et al. Risk factors for laparoscopically confirmed pelvic inflammatory disease: Findings from Mumbai (Bombay), India. *Sex Transm Infect.* 1998;74:426–32.
4. Gaitán H, Angel E, Medina M et al. Diagnóstico de la enfermedad pélvica inflamatoria en el Instituto Materno Infantil 1992–93. *Revista Facultad de Medicina, Universidad Nacional.* 1996;44:134–41.
5. Gaitán H, Angel E, Diaz R, Parada A, Sanchez L, Vargas C. Accuracy of five different diagnostic techniques in mild-to-moderate pelvic inflammatory disease. *Infect Dis Obstet Gynecol.* 2002;10:171–80.
6. Gaitan H, Angel E, Sánchez J et al. Laparoscopic diagnosis of acute lower abdominal pain in women of reproductive age. *Int J Obstet Gynecol.* 2002;76:149–58.
7. Paavonen J. Pelvic inflammatory disease: From diagnosis to prevention (a review). *Dermatol Clin.* 1998;16:747–56.
8. Molander P, Sjoberg J, Paavonen J, Cacciatore B. Transvaginal power Doppler findings in laparoscopically proven acute pelvic inflammatory disease. *Ultrasound Obstet Gynecol.* 2001;17:233–8.
9. Härkki-Sirén P, Kurki T. A nationwide analysis of laparoscopic complications. *Obstet Gynecol.* 1997;89:108–12.
10. Timor-Tritsch IE, Rottem S. Transvaginal ultrasonographic study of the fallopian tube. *Obstet Gynecol.* 1987;70:424–8.

11. Timor-Tritsch IE, Bar Yam Y, Elgali S, Rottem S. The technique of transvaginal sonography with the use of a 6.5 Mhz probe. *Am J Obstet Gynecol.* 1988;158:1019–24.

12. Tessler FN, Perrella RR, Fleischer AL, Grant EG. Endovaginal sonographic diagnosis of dilated Fallopian tubes. *Am J Roentgenol.* 1989;153:523–5.

13. Bulas DI, Ahlstrom PA, Sivit CJ, Blask ARN, ODonnell RM. Pelvic inflammatory disease in the adolescent: Comparison of transabdominal and transvaginal sonographic evaluation. *Radiology.* 1992;183:435–9.

14. Patten RM, Vincent LM, Wolner-Hanssen P, Thorpe E Jr. Pelvic inflammatory disease: Endovaginal sonography with laparoscopic correlation. *J Ultrasound Med.* 1990;9:681–9.

15. Cacciatore B, Leminen A, Ingman-Freiberg S, Ylostalo P, Paavonen J. Transvaginal sonographic findings in ambulatory patients with suspected pelvic inflammatory disease. *Obstet Gynecol.* 1992;80:912–16.

16. Atri M, Tran CN, Bret PM, Aldis AE, Kintzen GM. Accuracy of endovaginal sonography for the detection of fallopian tubes. *Am J Roentgenol.* 1989;153:523–5.

17. Taipale P, Tarjanne H, Ylöstalo P. Transvaginal sonography in suspected pelvic inflammatory disease. *Ultrasound Obstet Gynecol* 1995;6:430–4.

18. Timor-Tritsch IE, Rottem S, Lewitt N. "The fallopian tube." *Transvaginal Sonography,* 2nd ed. Timor-Tritsch IE, Rottem S (eds). New York. Chapman & Hall. 1991, pp. 131–44.

19. Bellah RD, Rosenberg HK. Transvaginal ultrasound in a children's hospital: Is it worthwhile? *Pediatr Radiol.* 1991;21:570–4.

20. Patel MD, Acord DL, Young SW. Likelihood ratio of sonographic findings in discriminating hydrosalpinx from other adnexal masses. *AJR Am J Roentgenol.* 2006 April;186:1033–8.

21. Timor-Tritsch IE. "Adnexal masses." *Ultrasound in Gynecology.* Goldstein SR, Timor-Tritsch IE (eds). New York. Churchill-Livingstone. 1995, pp. 103–14.

22. Timor-Tritsch IE, Lerner JP, Monteagudo A, Murphy KE, Heller DS. Transvaginal sonographic markers of tubal inflammatory disease. *Ultrasound Obstet Gynecol.* 1998;12:56–66.

23. Russin LD. Imaging of hydrosalpinx with torsion following tubal sterilization. *Semin Ultrasound CT MRI.* 1988;9:175–82.

24. Zeger W, Holt K. Gynecologic infections. *Emerg Med Clin N Am.* 2003;21:631–48.

25. Strouse PJ, DiPietro MA, Teo EL, Doi K, Chrisp CE. Power Doppler evaluation of joint effusions: Investigation in a rabbit model. *Pediatr Radiol.* 1999;29:617–23.

26. Arslan H, Sakarya ME, Bozkurt M, Unal O, Dilek ON, Harman M. The role of power Doppler sonography in the evaluation of suspected soft tissue abscesses. *Eur J Ultrasound.* 1998;8:101–6.

27. Hillis SD, Joesoef R, Marchbanks PA, Wasserheit JN, Cates W Jr, Westrom L. Delayed care of pelvic inflammatory disease as a risk factor of impaired infertility. *Am J Obstet Gynecol.* 1993;168:1503–9.

28. Pavletic AJ, Eschenbach DA, Wölner-Hanssen P, Paavonen J, Hawes SE, Holmes KK. Infertility following pelvic inflammatory disease. *Infect Dis Obstet Gynecol.* 1999;7:145–52.

29. Kurjak A, Kupesic S. Scoring system for the prediction of ovarian endometriosis based on transvaginal color and pulsed Doppler sonography. *Fertil Steril.* 1994;62:81–88.

30. Kupesic S, Kurjak A, Pasalic L, Benic S, Ilijas M. The value of transvaginal color Doppler in the assessment of pelvic inflammatory disease. *Ultrasound Med Biol.* 1995;21:733–8.

31. Alatas C, Aksoy E, Akarsu C, Yakin K, Bahceci M. Hemodynamic assessment in pelvic inflammatory disease by transvaginal color Doppler ultrasonography. *Eur J Obstet Gynecol.* 1996;70:75–78.

32. Tepper R, Aviram R, Cohen N, Cohen I, Holtzinger M, Beyth Y. Doppler flow characteristics in patients with pelvic inflammatory disease: Responders versus nonresponders to therapy. *J Clin Ultrasound.* 1998;26:247–9.

33. Guerriero S, Ajossa S, Lai MP, Risalvato A, Paoletti MP, Melis GB. Clinical applications of colour Doppler energy imaging in the female reproductive tract and pregnancy. *Hum Reprod Update.* 1999;5:515–29.

CHAPTER 5

Dysmenorrhea and Adenomyosis

Juan Luis Alcázar

INTRODUCTION

Dysmenorrhea is defined as the presence of painful cramps of uterine origin during menstruation and constitutes one of the most common problems in women of all ages and races.[1,2] The exact prevalence of dysmenorrhea is difficult to determine, but estimates vary widely ranging from 45% to 93% of women.[1]

There are some risk factors for dysmenorrhea such as heavy menstrual flow, premenstrual syndrome, irregular menstrual cycle, age (younger than 30 years old), menarche before 12 years old, and low body mass index.[2]

Dysmenorrhea is classified as primary dysmenorrhea (menstrual pain without organic disease) or secondary dysmenorrhea (menstrual pain associated with underlying pelvic pathology).[1] The most frequent causes of secondary dysmenorrhea are endometriosis and adenomyosis; other causes of secondary dysmenorrhea may be endometrial polyps, uterine myomas, uterine congenital anomalies, and pelvic inflammatory disease.[2]

In this chapter, we will review ultrasound findings related to primary dysmenorrhea and adenomyosis. Other causes of secondary dysmenorrhea are addressed in other chapters of this book.

PRIMARY DYSMENORRHEA

As stated earlier, primary dysmenorrhea is defined as menstrual pain without organic uterine or pelvic disease. Therefore, diagnosis is achieved after ruling out any kind of uterine or pelvic lesion. The ultimate cause of primary dysmenorrhea has not yet been determined. However, it is well known that an excessive level of uterine prostaglandins ($PGF2_{alpha}$ and $PGF2$) producing an increased uterine tone and high-amplitude contractions

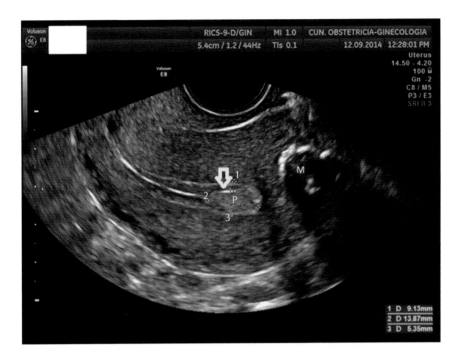

FIGURE 5.1   Transvaginal ultrasound showing an endometrial polyp as a hyperechoic, homogeneous, well-defined lesion (P) within the endometrium. The bright edge sign is visible (arrow). A calcified myoma is also seen (M).

play an important role in the pathogenesis of dysmenorrhea.[1] This higher activity of uterine muscle may lead to uterine ischemia and secondary pain.[3]

Ultrasound examination should be considered for all women presenting with primary dysmenorrhea,[1,2] since causes of secondary dysmenorrhea, such as endometrial polyps (Figure 5.1) or uterine myomas (Figure 5.2), should be ruled out before a diagnosis of primary dysmenorrhea is provided. Therefore, ultrasound evaluation of the uterus and adnexal should render normal results in women with primary dysmenorrhea (Figures 5.3 and 5.4). Pelvic examination should also be normal. Zebitay et al. reported that girls with severe dysmenorrhea had larger cervical length as assessed by transabdominal ultrasound than those without dysmenorrhea.[4] This is an interesting finding, but no other studies have confirmed it.

Because of the potential relationship of uterine ischemia and primary dysmenorrhea, some studies have evaluated uterine vascularization using Doppler ultrasound in women with primary dysmenorrhea. Dmitrovic et al. evaluated a case series of 42 women with primary dysmenorrhea and 50 healthy controls.[5] They found that pulsed Doppler indices (pulsatility and resistance indices) of the uterine and arcuate arteries were significantly higher (Figure 5.5) in women with dysmenorrhea as compared with controls, not only during menstruation but also during the whole menstrual cycle. These findings supported the idea of uterine ischemia as a mechanism involved in the pathogenesis of primary dysmenorrhea. Similar findings were reported by Altunyurt et al.[6]

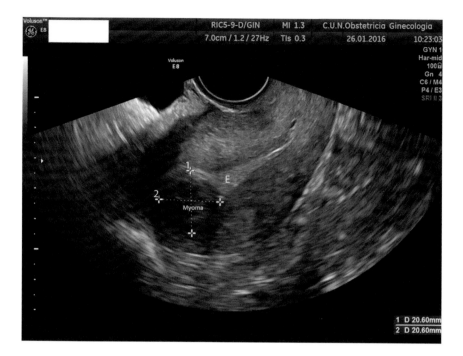

FIGURE 5.2 Transvaginal ultrasound showing a myoma as a hypoechoic, homogeneous, well-defined lesion within the myometrium, displacing the endometrium (E).

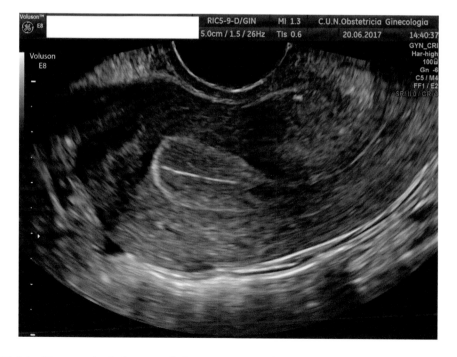

FIGURE 5.3 Transvaginal ultrasound showing a normal trilaminar endometrium (longitudinal plane) in a woman with primary dysmenorrhea.

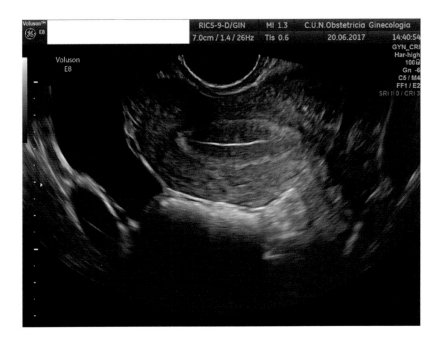

FIGURE 5.4   The same case as in Figure 5.3, a transverse plane.

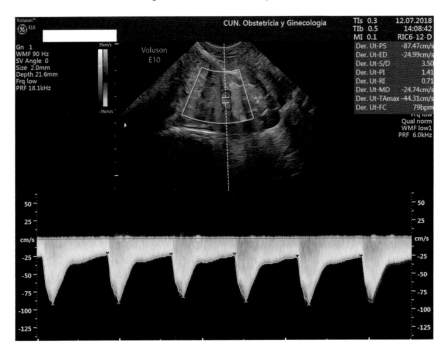

FIGURE 5.5   Flow velocity waveform assessed by pulsed Doppler of the uterine artery.

Dmitrovic et al. also found that severity of dysmenorrhea was related to pulsed Doppler indices from the arcuate arteries.[7] Women with severe dysmenorrhea had a higher resistance index (less blood flow) in the arcuate arteries during the luteal phase as compared to women with mild dysmenorrhea and controls. Interestingly, Celik et al. reported similar findings

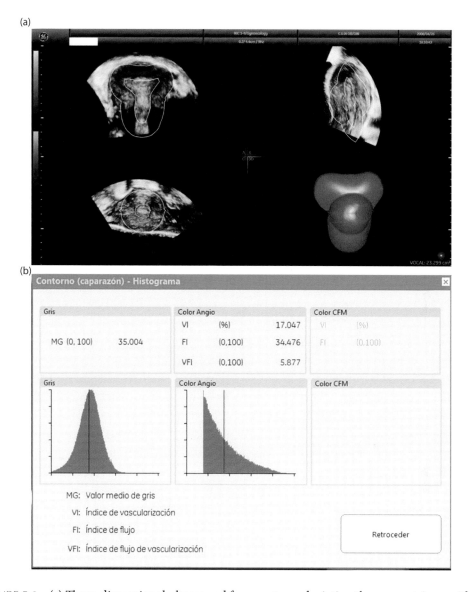

FIGURE 5.6 (a) Three-dimensional ultrasound from a uterus depicting the myometrium, with the (b) corresponding three-dimensional vascular indices.

to Dmitrovic et al.[8] However, Celik et al. found that uterine artery blood flow was reduced at night, reflecting a circadian change in uterine blood flow in women with primary dysmenorrhea. This was not the case for healthy controls.

Royo and Alcázar evaluated myometrial vascularization using three-dimensional power Doppler angiography in women with different grades of primary dysmenorrhea.[9] Using this technique, they evaluated the whole myometrial vascularization by calculating the three-dimensional power Doppler indices, namely, the vascularization index (VI), flow index (FI), and vascularization-flow index (VFI), at the moment of maximum pain as referred by the patients (Figure 5.6). They found that VI and VFI were significantly higher in women with severe dysmenorrhea as compared with women with mild or no dysmenorrhea. These findings were rather surprising since higher VI and VFI mean higher vascularization. The authors hypothesized that their findings could be explained by substantial venous ectasia of blood flow (power Doppler cannot discriminate between venous and arterial vessels) because of uterine muscle contraction.

In summary, the main role of ultrasound for assessing women with primary dysmenorrhea is to rule out the presence of uterine or pelvic pathology. There is some evidence that uterine blood flow might be reduced in women with severe primary dysmenorrhea supporting the idea that uterine ischemia is one of the mechanisms involved in the pathogenesis of primary dysmenorrhea.

ADENOMYOSIS

General Considerations

Adenomyosis is a uterine benign condition defined as the presence of endometrial glands in the myometrium.[10] Its etiology and pathogenesis are not yet fully understood. The prevalence has been estimated to be 20%–35% of women.[11,12] Risk factors for adenomyosis include multiparity, termination of pregnancy, cesarean section delivery, early menarche, obesity, short cycles, uterine curettage, and women's age.[11,12]

Definitive diagnosis of adenomyosis requires histological analysis.[11] Hysterectomy would be the best method. However, this is not so simple since many women with adenomyosis are in their reproductive age. Less invasive techniques, such as uterine needle biopsy, have been proposed showing high specificity but limited sensitivity.[13,14]

As stated earlier, the pathogenesis of adenomyosis is still not well known. There are two theories for explaining the origin of this disease. The one most commonly accepted states that adenomyosis results from the invagination of the endometrial basalis as a result of tissue injury and repair mechanism. There is also the theory that adenomyosis results from metaplasia of displaced embryonic pluripotent Müllerian remnants or differentiation of adult stem cells.[15]

There is no pathognomonic symptoms associated to adenomyosis. The most common symptoms related to adenomyosis are pelvic pain (dysmenorrhea, dyspareunia, or chromic pelvic pain), abnormal uterine bleeding, and feeling of swelling. However, up to 30% of women with adenomyosis are asymptomatic.[16,17] This spectrum of symptoms are nonspecific and may be present in other uterine and pelvic pathologies, such as endometriosis, uterine leiomyoma, or endometrial polyps.

Adenomyosis has been related to impaired fertility and poor pregnancy outcome.[16,18,19]

The treatment of adenomyosis depends on symptoms such as pain, abnormal uterine bleeding, and fertility problems. Medical therapy used to be first-line treatment for adenomyosis. There is a wide range of medical therapy options, but currently there is not a single drug labeled for adenomyosis. Furthermore, there are no specific guidelines to follow for the best management of adenomyosis.[20]

Among the different medical treatments, nonsteroidal anti-inflammatory drugs and hormonal therapy such as progestins (norethindrone acetate, danazol, dienogest, and levonorgestrel-releasing intrauterine system) or oral contraceptives are the most commonly used. GnRH analogues may also be an option. However, add-back therapy should be used.[20] There are some drugs under investigation, including aromatase inhibitors, selective progesterone receptor modulators, GnRH antagonists, valproic acid, and antiplatelet therapy.[20]

Surgery may also play a role for treating adenomyosis.[21,22] The indication for surgical treatment includes failure of medical therapy, infertility, recurrent miscarriage, and desire to preserve fertility. Total hysterectomy is the gold standard for surgical treatment.[21] This procedure is considered as the definitive treatment success, for bleeding symptoms relief is 100%, but there is a chance for persistence of pain (especially if endometriosis also exists). The chance of symptoms recurrence almost does not exist. However, preservation of fertility is not possible.[21] As an alternative to hysterectomy, some other techniques have been proposed, such as adenomyomectomy, wedge resection of the uterine wall, wedge-shaped uterine wall removal, triple-flap technique, and asymmetric dissection technique.[22]

Ultrasound Diagnosis of Adenomyosis

The spectrum of findings related to adenomyosis is wide. Before describing ultrasound findings, it is important to discuss the classification of adenomyosis. There have been several attempts for classifying the types and extension of adenomyosis based on ultrasound, magnetic resonance imaging, and clinical histological findings (Table 5.1).[16]

Transvaginal ultrasound (TVS) has been reported as a good imaging technique for assessing uterine adenomyosis.[23] When assessing adenomyosis by transvaginal ultrasound, it is important to take into account that the myometrium has three distinct sonographic layers: the outer, the middle, and the inner. The inner layer is just beneath the endometrium, and it is seen as hypoechogenic on the transvaginal ultrasound and referred to as the junctional zone (JZ). The middle layer is the most echogenic and is separated from the outer layer by the arcuate vessels, and the outer layer extends from the arcuate vessels to the uterine serosa (Figure 5.7).[23]

There are several ultrasonographic criteria associated to adenomyosis, including a globally enlarged uterus (Figure 5.8), presence of fan-shaped shadowing (Figure 5.9), myometrial asymmetry (Figure 5.10), echogenic islands within the myometrium (Figure 5.11), myometrial cysts (Figure 5.12), thickening of the JZ (Figure 5.13), interrupted or irregular JZ (Figure 5.14), and heterogeneous myometrium (Figure 5.15).[23–25]

Most adenomyotic lesions are ill-defined. However, in some circumstances they may be better circumscribed and demonstrate mass effect, the so-called adenomyomas (Figure 5.16). Although adenomyomas may seem well defined, the ectopic endometrial tissue is often more diffuse within the myometrium.[24] Myometrial cysts may vary in number, size, and location (Figure 5.17).

Color or power Doppler may help for diagnosing adenomyosis, since an increased focal vascularization may be observed (Figure 5.18) and for discriminating adenomyomas from leiomyomas, since vessels appear perpendicular to endometrium in adenomyosis, whereas they appear as surrounding the lesion in case of leiomyomas (Figure 5.19).[23,25]

The JZ can be observed by two-dimensional ultrasound.[23] However, three-dimensional ultrasound has emerged as a new technique that allows a better assessment of the JZ, especially of the JZ in the coronal plane. Exacoustos et al. found that JZ thickness as well as JZ disruption were associated to the presence of adenomyosis.[26] They proposed measuring the JZ on the

TABLE 5.1   Classifications of the Types and Extension of Adenomyosis

Author	Year	Classification	Criteria
Bird[47]	1972	Grade I: Subbasal endometrium Grade II: Up to mid myometrium Grade III: Beyond mid myometrium	Histology
Gordts[48]	2008	JZ hyperplasia (JZ thickness 8–12 mm) 　Partial 　Diffuse Adenomyosis with JZ >12 mm involving the outer myometrium 　with glandular foci Adenomyomas (myometrial masses with indistinct margins)	MRI
Kishi[49]	2012	Type I (intrinsic): Adenomyosis involving the JZ Type II (extrinsic): Adenomyosis affects the outer shell of the uterus 　but not the inner Type III (intramural): Adenomyosis affects only the myometrium Type IV (indeterminate): Findings not classifiable according to 　types I–III	MRI
Chapron[50]	2017	Isolated diffuse adenomyosis Isolated focal adenomyosis involving the outer myometrium (FAOM) Associated diffuse and FAOM adenomyosis	MRI
Pistofidis[51]	2014	Diffuse Sclerotic Nodular Cystic	Histology
Grimbizis	2014[52]	Diffuse: Including JZ thickening and outer myometrium extensive 　disease Focal: Including adenomyomas and cystic adenomyosis Polypoid adenomyomas 　Typical 　Atypical Other forms 　Adenomyoma of endocervical type 　Retroperitoneal adenomyomas	Histology
Bazot	2018[25]	Internal adenomyosis 　Focal 　Superficial 　Diffuse 　Adenomyomas External adenomyosis 　Posterior 　Anterior	MRI

coronal and longitudinal planes of the uterus at the level of the maximum and minimum thickness (Figure 5.20). They found that a maximum thickness of JZ $\geq$8 mm or a difference between maximum and minimum thickness of $\geq$4 mm were highly predictive of adenomyosis. Luciano et al. reported similar results.[27] Interestingly, these authors reported that diagnostic accuracy of three-dimensional ultrasound for assessing JZ decreased significantly in patients who had previously undergone endometrial ablation or in women receiving medical therapy.

Recently, a classification and reporting system for diagnosing adenomyosis has been proposed.[28] This proposal is based on the identification of adenomyosis according to the

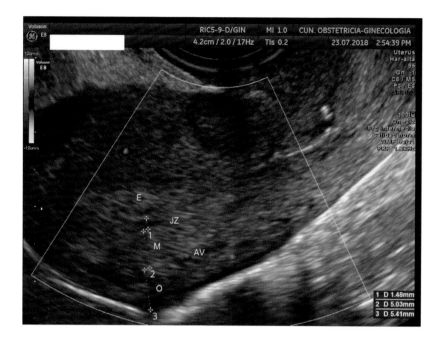

FIGURE 5.7 Transvaginal ultrasound depicting the layers of the myometrium. JZ, junctional zone (observed as a hypoechoic line); M, middle layer; O, outer layer; AV, arcuate vessels; E, endometrium.

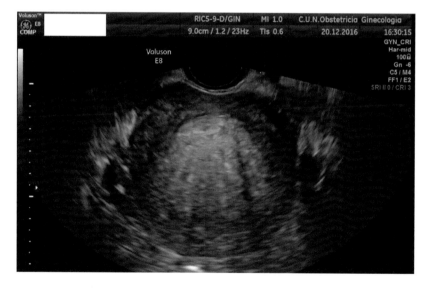

FIGURE 5.8 Transvaginal ultrasound depicting a globally enlarged uterus in a case of adenomyosis. Fan-shaped shadowing is also present.

Morphological Uterus Sonographic Assessment (MUSA) criteria (Table 5.2),[29] disease location (anterior, posterior, left lateral, right lateral, fundal), type of lesion (diffuse or focal), presence of intralesional cysts, myometrial layer involvement (junctional zone, myometrium, serosa), disease extent (<25%, 25%–50%, >50% of uterine volume affected by adenomyosis), and lesion size.

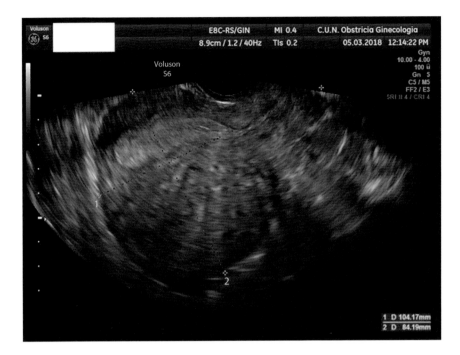

FIGURE 5.9   Transvaginal ultrasound depicting fan-shaped shadowing in an adenomyotic uterus.

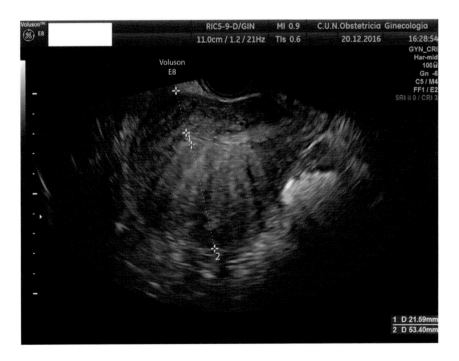

FIGURE 5.10   Transvaginal ultrasound depicting a myometrial asymmetry (anterior wall: 21.6 mm, posterior wall: 53.4 mm) in a case of adenomyosis.

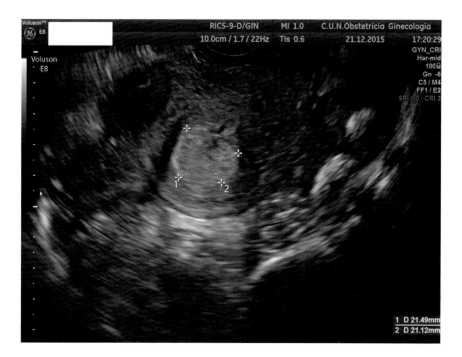

FIGURE 5.11   Transvaginal ultrasound depicting a myometrial echogenic island in a case of adenomyosis.

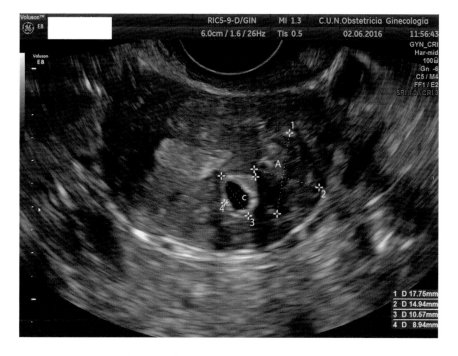

FIGURE 5.12   Transvaginal ultrasound depicting a myometrial cyst with echogenic rim (c) and an adenomyoma (A), shown as an ill-defined heterogeneous lesion, in a case of adenomyosis.

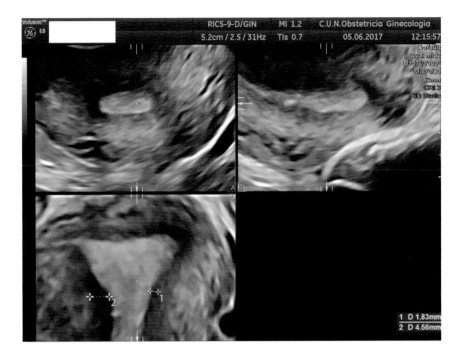

FIGURE 5.13   Measurement of junctional zone (JZ) thickness using 3D ultrasound with volume contrast imaging (VCI). Note the thickening of the JZ in the right lateral uterine wall.

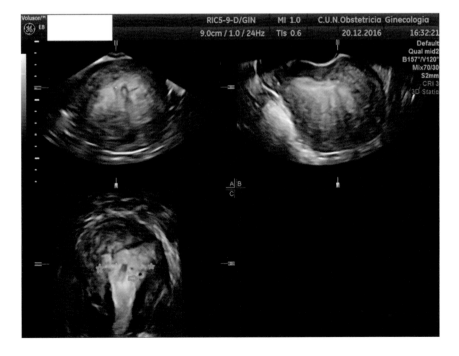

FIGURE 5.14   Three-dimensional ultrasound depicting an interrupted junctional zone in the uterine coronal plane (asterisks). A cystic lesion in the JZ is also observed (arrow).

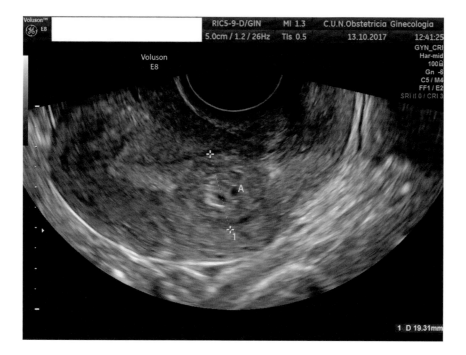

FIGURE 5.15   Transvaginal ultrasound depicting a heterogeneous myometrium in a case of adenomyosis. It seems that there is also adenomyoma (A), shown as an ill-defined heterogeneous lesion.

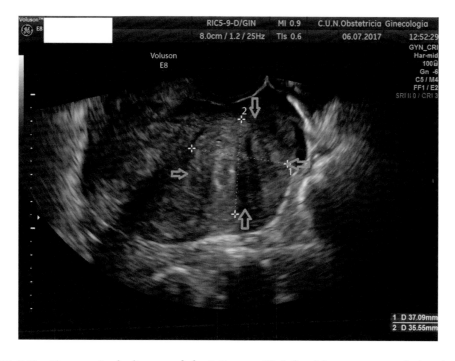

FIGURE 5.16   Transvaginal ultrasound depicting an ill-defined heterogeneous lesion (arrows) described as adenomyoma in a case of adenomyosis.

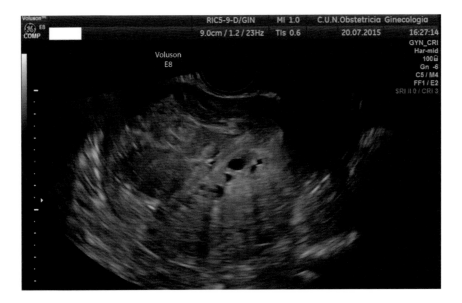

FIGURE 5.17 Transvaginal ultrasound depicting myometrial cysts in the posterior uterine wall. As it may be observed, size among the cysts varies.

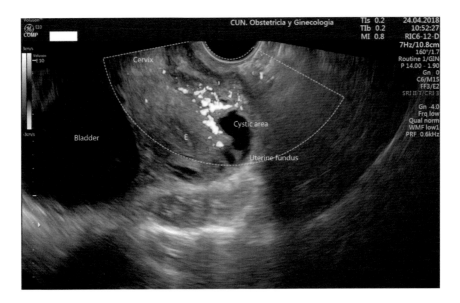

FIGURE 5.18 Transvaginal ultrasound showing a focal increased myometrial vascularization in a case of adenomyosis. E, endometrium.

Some authors have stated that the diagnosis of adenomyosis should be based on the presence of at least three of these criteria.[23] However, this has been challenged by others.[25]

Other researchers have reported that the number of ultrasound features seen during TVS is related to the severity of dysmenorrhea associated to adenomyosis.[30] However, many of the ultrasound features associated to adenomyosis are based on the examiner's subjective impression. Therefore, reproducibility is a relevant issue. However, there are

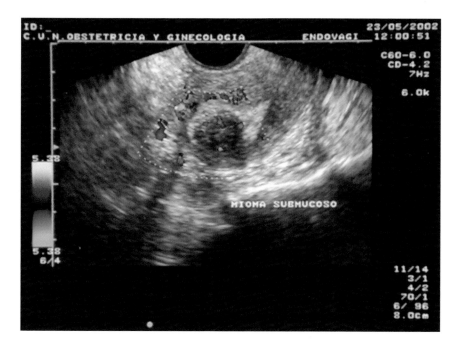

FIGURE 5.19   Transvaginal ultrasound showing the typical round vascularization in a myoma. This may help to discriminate between myoma and adenomyoma.

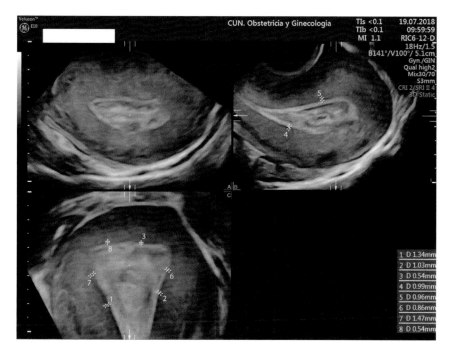

FIGURE 5.20   Measurement of junctional zone (JZ) thickness using 3D ultrasound with volume contrast imaging (VCI) as proposed by Exacoustos et al.[26]

TABLE 5.2   Ultrasound Criteria for Diagnosing Ultrasound

Ultrasound Feature	Adenomyosis
Serosal contour of the uterus	Globally enlarged uterus
Definition of the lesion	Ill-defined in diffuse adenomyosis Adenomyoma may be well defined
Symmetry of uterine walls	Myometrial anteroposterior asymmetry
Lesion outline	Ill-defined
Lesion shape	Ill-defined
Lesion contour	Irregular or ill-defined
Lesion rim	No rim
Lesion shadowing	Fan-shaped shadowing No edge shadows
Lesion echogenicity	Nonuniform Mixed Cystic areas or lacunae Subendometrial lines and buds
Lesion vascularity	Translesional blond flow
JZ	Thickened, irregular, or ill-defined Interrupted

scanty data about reproducibility of ultrasound features among different observers. Puente et al. reported a good agreement among expert observers for diagnosing adenomyosis using three-dimensional ultrasound volumes when at least one feature was present.[31] However, interobserver agreement for each specific feature analyzed (globular uterus, myometrial asymmetry, myometrial heterogeneity, myometrial cysts, disrupted JZ) was moderate.[31]

Regarding the reproducibility of JZ visualization and thickness measurement, Naftalin et al. reported good inter- and intraobserver agreement for JZ visualizations. Parity and endometrial thickness significantly affect visualization: the larger endometrial thickness, the better visualization; and the higher parity, the poorer visualization.[32] More recently, Rasmussen et al. showed that repeatability and reliability of JZ measurements between expert and nonexpert examiners is poor with measurement errors ranging from ± 2 to ± 4 mm.[33]

Several meta-analyses have been reported addressing the diagnostic performance of TVS for diagnosing adenomyosis. Meredith et al. reported a meta-analysis including 14 studies comprising 1895 women. They reported a pooled sensitivity and specificity for TVS of 82.5% and 84.6%, respectively.[34] However, these authors did not assess diagnostic performance of specific ultrasound features and did not include three-dimensional ultrasound studies. Champaneria et al. reported another systematic review including 23 studies comprising 2312 women. Pooled sensitivity and specificity for TVS were 72% and 81%, respectively. However, they did not assess diagnostic performance of specific ultrasound features.[35] Dartmouth reported a meta-analysis including nine studies involving 1302 patients. However, the heterogeneity found between studies was so great that it precluded statistical data pooling.[36] The most recent meta-analysis has been reported by Andres et al.[37] These authors included eight studies involving 763 women. They included studies using two-dimensional and three-dimensional ultrasound, and histological analysis after hysterectomy as a reference standard. They reported the diagnostic performance for some specific ultrasound features (Table 5.3).

TABLE 5.3   Diagnostic Performance of Ultrasound Features for Diagnosing Adenomyosis

Ultrasound Feature	Pooled Sensitivity (%)		Pooled Specificity (%)	
	2D	3D	2D	3D
Myometrial wall asymmetry	57.2	59.2	71.9	53.4
Myometrial cysts	72	58.2	62.7	54.3
Heterogeneous myometrium	86	82.7	61.3	41.4
Fan-shaped shadowing	71.3	—	79.7	—
Disruption JZ	58.6	87.8	71.5	56.0
Globular uterus	55	—	80.2	—

Elastography is a new ultrasound-based technique that allows the assessment of tissue stiffness. There are two main forms of ultrasound elastography: strain elastography and shear wave elastography.[38] Some studies have addressed the role of elastography for diagnosing adenomyosis. Tessarolo et al., using strain elastography, found that adenomyotic lesions presented more softness as compared to surrounding normal uterine tissue (Figure 5.21).[39] Frank et al., also using strain elastography, reported that this technique could be useful for discriminating adenomyoma from leiomyoma, since strain measurements were lower in adenomyoma than in leiomyoma.[40] They also reported that repeatability of strain measurement was good. Acar et al. reported on the use of shear wave elastography. They also found that stiffness was significantly increased in adenomyotic lesions.[38] More recently, Stoelinga et al. reported that elastography may be useful for discriminating adenomyomas from uterine fibroids, with high agreement between different observers.[41]

Role of MRI in the Diagnosis of Adenomyosis

Magnetic resonance imaging is considered as a second-line imaging technique for diagnosing uterine adenomyosis, mainly when ultrasound evaluation in not conclusive.[25] Most studies reported comparing TVS and MRI show that MRI did not significantly provide better diagnostic performance than TVS, but may help in some cases since it is more specific.[25,35,42] MRI may be considered as less operator-dependent than TVS, but expertise is required.[25]

Summary

Adenomyosis is a relatively common benign uterine disease causing pelvic pain, abnormal uterine bleeding, and fertility problems. Transvaginal ultrasound is considered as the first-line imaging technique for diagnosing adenomyosis. There is a wide spectrum of sonographic findings associated with adenomyosis. Three-dimensional ultrasound allows the assessment of the uterine junctional zone. The most sensitive ultrasound features are the heterogeneous myometrium on two-dimensional ultrasound and disruption of the JZ on three-dimensional ultrasound. The most specific finding in the presence of a globular uterus. New ultrasound techniques such as elastography may have a role in the future. MRI is the second-line imaging technique and may be a problem-solving technique in many circumstances.

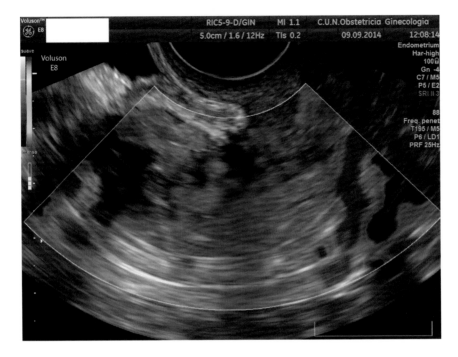

FIGURE 5.21   Elastography from a normal uterus. In color scale from blue to red means from harder to softer tissue.

There is a need for more and better designed studies assessing the interobserver agreement and learning curve for transvaginal ultrasound evaluation of adenomyosis. Additionally, there is a need for a consensus for reporting ultrasound findings in adenomyosis.

SECONDARY DYSMENORRHEA

Secondary dysmenorrhea refers to dysmenorrhea caused by some pathological entities. The most common forms are adenomyosis (see earlier), endometriosis (see Chapter 2), and uterine myomas or endometrial polyps (see earlier). However, there may be other, less common causes of secondary dysmenorrhea, such as intrauterine synechiae, displaced intrauterine devices, and intratubal devices (Essure®).

Intrauterine Synechiae

Intrauterine synechiae, also termed Asherman syndrome, is characterized by the formation of adhesions in the uterine cavity.[43] The characteristic findings at transvaginal ultrasound are irregular endometrium, interruption of the endometrial lining at the site of adhesions (Figure 5.22), echogenic endometrium, and echolucent areas.[44] However, the sensitivity and specificity for transvaginal ultrasound are low (52% and 11%, respectively). Sonohysterography offers a better diagnostic performance (100% accuracy), but hysteroscopy is considered as the gold standard technique for diagnosing intrauterine synechiae.[45]

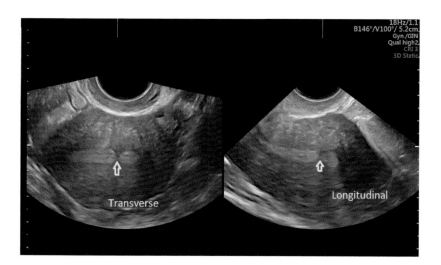

FIGURE 5.22   Transvaginal ultrasound showing a case of Asherman syndrome. An interruption of the endometrial lining is seen at the site of the adhesion (arrows).

Intrauterine Device Displacement

Intrauterine device displacement constitutes a common complication of both conventional intrauterine devices (IUDs) and intratubal devices.[46] Displacement may consist of explusion, simple displacement or migration, and perforation. Three-dimensional ultrasound has been proved a better technique than two-dimensional ultrasound for assessing displaced IUDs or Essure devices,[46] especially for the assessment of the coronal plane (Figures 5.23 through 5.25).

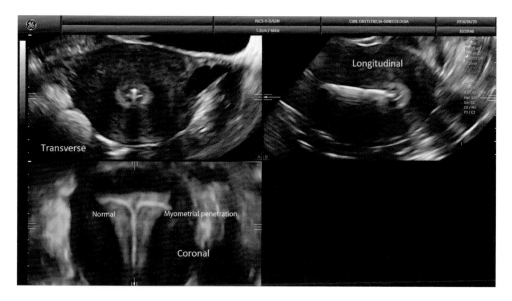

FIGURE 5.23   Three-dimensional ultrasound showing a case of partial myometrial penetration of an IUD in a woman presenting with secondary dysmenorrhea several months after IUD insertion. Note the coronal plane.

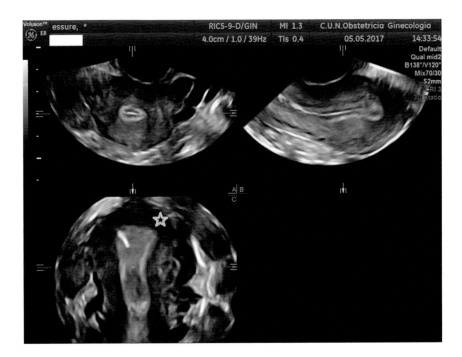

FIGURE 5.24   Three-dimensional ultrasound showing a case of a woman presenting with secondary dysmenorrhea and chronic pelvic pain several months after Essure insertion. In the coronal plane, the device can be observed on one side, but on the other side the device is missing (asterisk), suspecting perforation and migration to the pelvic cavity, confirmed at laparoscopic assessment.

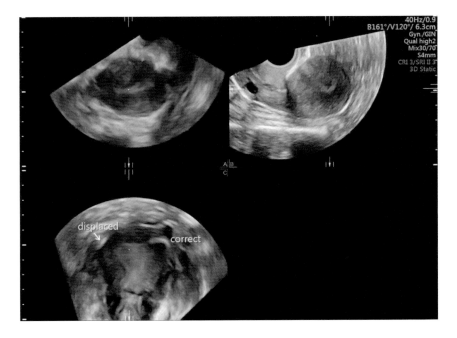

FIGURE 5.25   Three-dimensional ultrasound showing a case of a woman presenting with secondary dysmenorrhea several months after Essure insertion. In the coronal plane, the device can be observed correctly placed and displaced.

REFERENCES

1. Bernardi M, Lazzeri L, Perelli F, Reis FM, Petraglia F. Dysmenorrhea and related disorders. *F1000Research.* 2017;6:1645.

2. Osayande AS, Mehulic S. Diagnosis and initial management of dysmenorrhea. *Am Fam Physician.* 2014;89:341–6.

3. Akerlund M. Vascularization of human endometrium. Uterine blood flow in healthy condition and in primary dysmenorrhoea. *Ann NY Acad Sci.* 1994;734:47–56.

4. Zebitay AG, Verit FF, Sakar MN, Keskin S, Cetin O, Ulusoy AI. Importance of cervical length in dysmenorrhoea aetiology. *J Obstet Gynaecol.* 2016;36:540–3.

5. Dmitrovic R. Transvaginal color Doppler study of uterine blood flow in primary dysmenorrhea. *Acta Obstet Gynecol Scand.* 2000;79:1112–6.

6. Altunyurt S, Göl M, Altunyurt S, Sezer O, Demir N. Primary dysmenorrhea and uterine blood flow: A color Doppler study. *J Reprod Med.* 2005;50:251–5.

7. Dmitrovic R, Peter B, Cvitkovic-Kuzmic A, Strelec M, Kereshi T. Severity of symptoms in primary dysmenorrhea—A Doppler study. *Eur J Obstet Gynecol Reprod Biol.* 2003;107:191–4.

8. Celik H, Gurates B, Parmaksiz C, Polat A, Hanay F, Kavak B, Yavuz A, Artas ZD. Severity of pain and circadian changes in uterine artery blood flow in primary dysmenorrhea. *Arch Gynecol Obstet.* 2009;280:589–92.

9. Royo P, Alcázar JL. Three-dimensional power Doppler assessment of uterine vascularization in women with primary dysmenorrhea. *J Ultrasound Med.* 2008;27:1003–10.

10. Donnez J, Donnez O, Dolmans MM. Introduction: Uterine adenomyosis, another enigmatic disease of our time. *Fertil Steril.* 2018;109:369–70.

11. Abbott JA. Adenomyosis and Abnormal Uterine Bleeding (AUB-A)—Pathogenesis, diagnosis, and management. *Best Pract Res Clin Obstet Gynaecol.* 2017;40:68–81.

12. Di Donato N, Montanari G, Benfenati A, Leonardi D, Bertoldo V, Monti G, Raimondo D, Seracchioli R. Prevalence of adenomyosis in women undergoing surgery for endometriosis. *Eur J Obstet Gynecol Reprod Biol.* 2014;181:289–93.

13. Brosens JJ, Barker FG. The role of myometrial needle biopsies in the diagnosis of adenomyosis. *Fertil Steril.* 1995;63:1347–9.

14. Vercellini P, Cortesi I, De Giorgi O, Merlo D, Carinelli SG, Crosignani PG. Transvaginal ultrasonography versus uterine needle biopsy in the diagnosis of diffuse adenomyosis. *Hum Reprod.* 1998;13:2884–7.

15. García-Solares J, Donnez J, Donnez O, Dolmans MM. Pathogenesis of uterine adenomyosis: Invagination or metaplasia? *Fertil Steril.* 2018;109:371–9.

16. Gordts S, Grimbizis G, Campo R. Symptoms and classification of uterine adenomyosis, including the place of hysteroscopy in diagnosis. *Fertil Steril.* 2018;109:380–88.e1.

17. Peric H, Fraser IS. The symptomatology of adenomyosis. *Best Pract Res Clin Obstet Gynaecol.* 2006;20:547–55.

18. Puente JM, Fabris A, Patel J, Patel A, Cerrillo M, Requena A, Garcia-Velasco JA. Adenomyosis in infertile women: Prevalence and the role of 3D ultrasound as a marker of severity of the disease. *Reprod Biol Endocrinol.* 2016;14:60.

19. Dueholm M. Uterine adenomyosis and infertility, review of reproductive outcome after in vitro fertilization and surgery. *Acta Obstet Gynecol Scand.* 2017;96:715–26.

20. Vannuccini S, Luisi S, Tosti C, Sorbi F, Petraglia F. Role of medical therapy in the management of uterine adenomyosis. *Fertil Steril.* 2018;109:398–405.

21. Oliveira MAP, Crispi CP Jr, Brollo LC, Crispi CP, De Wilde RL. Surgery in adenomyosis. *Arch Gynecol Obstet.* 2018;297:581–9.

22. Osada H. Uterine adenomyosis and adenomyoma: The surgical approach. *Fertil Steril.* 2018;109:406–17.

23. Dueholm M. Transvaginal ultrasound for diagnosis of adenomyosis: A review. *Best Pract Res Clin Obstet Gynaecol.* 2006;20:569–82.

24. Van den Bosch T, Van Schoubroeck D. Ultrasound diagnosis of endometriosis and adenomyosis: State of the art. *Best Pract Res Clin Obstet Gynaecol.* 2018;51:16–24.

25. Bazot M, Daraï E. Role of transvaginal sonography and magnetic resonance imaging in the diagnosis of uterine adenomyosis. *Fertil Steril.* 2018;109:389–397.

26. Exacoustos C, Brienza L, Di Giovanni A, Szabolcs B, Romanini ME, Zupi E, Arduini D. Adenomyosis: Three-dimensional sonographic findings of the junctional zone and correlation with histology. *Ultrasound Obstet Gynecol.* 2011;37:471–9.

27. Luciano DE, Exacoustos C, Albrecht L, LaMonica R, Proffer A, Zupi E, Luciano AA. Three-dimensional ultrasound in diagnosis of adenomyosis: Histologic correlation with ultrasound targeted biopsies of the uterus. *J Minim Invasive Gynecol.* 2013;20:803–10.

28. Van den Bosch T, de Bruijn AM, de Leeuw RA, Dueholm M, Exacoustos C, Valentin L, Bourne T, Timmerman D, Huirne JAF. A sonographic classification and reporting system for diagnosing adenomyosis. *Ultrasound Obstet Gynecol.* 2018 May 22.

29. Van den Bosch T, Dueholm M, Leone FP et al. Terms, definitions and measurements to describe sonographic features of myometrium and uterine masses: A consensus opinion from the Morphological Uterus Sonographic Assessment (MUSA) group. *Ultrasound Obstet Gynecol.* 2015;46:284–98.

30. Naftalin J, Hoo W, Nunes N, Holland T, Mavrelos D, Jurkovic D. Association between ultrasound features of adenomyosis and severity of menstrual pain. *Ultrasound Obstet Gynecol.* 2016;47:779–83.

31. Puente JM, Alcázar JL, Martinez-Ten MP, Bermejo C, Troncoso, MT, Garcia-Velasco JA. Interobserver agreement in the study of 2D and 3D sonographic criteria for adenomyosis. *J Endometr Pelvic Pain Disord.* 2017;9:211–215.

32. Naftalin J, Hoo W, Pateman K, Mavrelos D, Holland T, Jurkovic D. How common is adenomyosis? A prospective study of prevalence using transvaginal ultrasound in a gynaecology clinic. *Hum Reprod.* 2012;27:3432–9.

33. Rasmussen CK, Glavind J, Madsen LD, Uldbjerg N, Dueholm M. Repeatability of junctional zone measurements using 3-dimensional transvaginal sonography in healthy fertile women. *J Ultrasound Med.* 2016;35:1497–508.

34. Meredith SM, Sanchez-Ramos L, Kaunitz AM. Diagnostic accuracy of transvaginal sonography for the diagnosis of adenomyosis: Systematic review and metaanalysis. *Am J Obstet Gynecol.* 2009;201:107.e1–6.

35. Champaneria R, Abedin P, Daniels J, Balogun M, Khan KS. Ultrasound scan and magnetic resonance imaging for the diagnosis of adenomyosis: Systematic review comparing test accuracy. *Acta Obstet Gynecol Scand.* 2010;89:1374–84.

36. Dartmouth K. A systematic review with meta-analysis: The common sonographic characteristics of adenomyosis. *Ultrasound.* 2014;22:148–57.

37. Andres MP, Borrelli GM, Ribeiro J, Baracat EC, Abrão MS, Kho RM. Transvaginal ultrasound for the diagnosis of adenomyosis: Systematic review and meta-analysis. *J Minim Invasive Gynecol.* 2018;25:257–64.

38. Acar S, Millar E, Mitkova M, Mitkov V. Value of ultrasound shear wave elastography in the diagnosis of adenomyosis. *Ultrasound.* 2016;24:205–13.

39. Tessarolo M, Bonino L, Camanni M, Deltetto F. Elastosonography: A possible new tool for diagnosis of adenomyosis? *Eur Radiol.* 2011;21:1546–52.

40. Frank ML, Schäfer SD, Möllers M et al. Importance of transvaginal elastography in the diagnosis of uterine fibroids and adenomyosis. *Ultraschall Med.* 2016;37:373–8.

41. Stoelinga B, Hehenkamp WJK, Nieuwenhuis LL, Conijn MMA, van Waesberghe JHTM, Brölmann HAM, Huirne JAF. Accuracy and reproducibility of sonoelastography for the assessment of fibroids and adenomyosis, with magnetic resonance imaging as reference standard. *Ultrasound Med Biol.* 2018;44:1654–63.

42. Dueholm M, Lundorf E. Transvaginal ultrasound or MRI for diagnosis of adenomyosis. *Curr Opin Obstet Gynecol*. 2007;19:505–12.

43. Salazar CA, Isaacson K, Morris S. A comprehensive review of Asherman's syndrome: Causes, symptoms and treatment options. *Curr Opin Obstet Gynecol*. 2017;29:249–56.

44. Deans R, Abbott J. Review of intrauterine adhesions. *J Minim Invasive Gynecol*. 2010;17:555–69.

45. Salle B, Gaucherand P, de Saint Hilaire P, Rudigoz RC. Transvaginal sonohysterographic evaluation of intrauterine adhesions. *J Clin Ultrasound*. 1999;27:131–4.

46. Boortz HE, Margolis DJ, Ragavendra N, Patel MK, Kadell BM. Migration of intrauterine devices: Radiologic findings and implications for patient care. *Radiographics*. 2012;32:335–52.

47. Bird CC, McElin TW, Manalo-Estrella P. The elusive adenomyosis of the uterus—revisited. *Am J Obstet Gynecol*. 1972;112:583–93.

48. Gordts S, Brosens JJ, Fusi L, Benagiano G, Brosens I. Uterine adenomyosis: A need for uniform terminology and consensus classification. *Reprod Biomed Online*. 2008;17:244–8.

49. Kishi Y, Suginami H, Kuramori R, Yabuta M, Suginami R, Taniguchi F. Four subtypes of adenomyosis assessed by magnetic resonance imaging and their specification. *Am J Obstet Gynecol*. 2012;207:114.e1–7.

50. Chapron C, Tosti C, Marcellin L, Bourdon M, Lafay-Pillet MC, Millischer AE, Streuli I, Borghese B, Petraglia F, Santulli P. Relationship between the magnetic resonance imaging appearance of adenomyosis and endometriosis phenotypes. *Hum Reprod*. 2017;32:1393–1401.

51. Pistofidis G, Makrakis E, Koukoura O, Bardis N, Balinakos P, Anaf V. Distinct types of uterine adenomyosis based on laparoscopic and histopathologic criteria. *Clin Exp Obstet Gynecol*. 2014;41:113–8.

52. Grimbizis GF, Mikos T, Tarlatzis B. Uterus-sparing operative treatment for adenomyosis. *Fertil Steril*. 2014;101:472–87.

CHAPTER 6

Uterine Myoma

Stefano Guerriero, Silvia Ajossa, Alba Piras, Eleonora Musa, Virginia Zanda, Valerio Mais, and Anna Maria Paoletti

INTRODUCTION

Uterine fibroids (also known as leiomyomas or myomas) are the most common type of benign uterine tumors that originate from the myometrium, and are made of extracellular matrix with collagen, fibronectin, and proteoglycans.[1]

This kind of lesion is common in patients of reproductive age, with an estimated prevalence of up to 80% by the age of 50 years.[2]

The precise cause of fibroid growth is actually unknown. However, several risk factors are associated with their growth, such as age (>40, the frequency up to 60%–80%), inheritance, body mass index (maybe related to peripheral conversion of androgens to estrogens), race (Blacks RR 2–3, > Caucasians > Asians), infertility, alcohol intake, uterine infection (for myometrial injury, which can represent a predisposing factor), and early menarche. Premenopausal and postmenopausal women have the same incidence of myomas, but in the premenopausal period the woman more frequently has multiple and larger myomas compared to postmenopausal women; this likely happens because in the postmenopausal period there is a decrease in estrogen secretion and a myoma's growth generally stops.[3]

Clinical presentation of fibroids is highly related to their location, size, and number. About 50%–80% of myomas are asymptomatic. When symptomatic, they can induce abnormal uterine bleeding (AUB), discomfort and bloating, dysmenorrhea, dyspareunia, pelvic/abdominal pressure and acute pain, infertility, obstetric complications (such as miscarriage), and intra- and postpartum issues. AUB alone occurs in 30% of patients with myomas, in which there is an increase in the volume of menstrual blood (menorrhagia) corresponding to the number of myomas present, especially in case of subserosal fibroids.[4]

Very rarely, fibroids can cause acute complications, which manifest themselves mainly with acute pelvic pain. The most frequent complications of myomas are acute torsion of a subserosal pedunculated fibroma, acute urinary retention that can induce renal failure, red degeneration mainly during pregnancy, thromboembolism, mesenteric vein thrombosis, and intestinal necrosis.[5] These conditions enter in differential diagnosis with twisted adnexa, rupture of ovarian cyst, hemorrhagic corpus luteum, or ectopic pregnancy.[5] Pelvic or abdominal pressure is related to the myoma's size with associated urinary symptoms (urine retention and urinary frequency) due to tension on the bladder or intestinal symptoms (bowel obstruction, tenesmus, constipation) due to tension on the bowel. Moreover, it is important to evaluate purulence associated with pain, because these two symptoms may be due to an infection (pyomyoma).[6]

The natural history of fibroids includes degeneration, which occurs generally in cases of rapid growth when the blood supply is not sufficient. We can distinguish the following types of myoma degeneration:

1. Red degeneration (in almost two-thirds of all myomas), which is caused by acute infarction of the lesion, typical of pregnancy.

2. Hyaline degeneration (which occurs in about 65% of myomas), characterized by the substitution of the degenerated tissue with fibrous tissue.

3. Myxomatous degeneration (in 15% of the cases).

4. Calcification, in 10% of the cases.

5. Cystic and fatty degeneration, rare.

6. Malignant degeneration, which occurs in less than 1/1000 cases.[3]

Based on location, the European Society for Gynecological Endoscopy (ESGE) proposed a very simple classification:

- G0 refers to a pedunculated intrauterine fibroma.

- G1 is a fibroma that grows more than 50% of its mass in the uterine cavity.

- G2 is a fibroma that grows more than 50% of its mass in the myometrial wall.[1]

The FIGO (International Federation of Gynecology and Obstetrics) classification, published by Munro et al. in 2011, describes eight types of fibroids and includes association of two types of myomas (Figure 6.1).[21] In clinical practice, distinct types of myomas may be present at the same time, and the FIGO classification better represents a realistic "map" of myoma localization.[1]

ULTRASOUND ASSESSMENT OF UTERINE MYOMAS

The ultrasonographic (US) evaluation of myomas is currently considered an easy, cost-effective, and accurate diagnostic method using the transvaginal and/or transabdominal probe.[7]

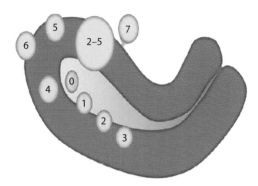

FIGURE 6.1   FIGO classifications of myomas locations adapted by Munro et al. Fibroid types range from 0 to 8. 0 = Pedunculated, intracavitary; 1 = Submucosal, <50% intramural; 2 = Submucosal, ≥50% intramural; 3 = Contact with endometrium, 100% intramural; 4 = Intramural; 5 = Subserosal, ≥50% intramural; 6 = Subserosal, <50% intramural; 7 = Subserosal, pedunculated; 8 = Other (e.g., cervical, parasitic). Where two numbers are given (e.g., 2–5), the first number refers to the relationship with the endometrium and the second number refers to the relationship with the serosa. For example, 2–5 means submucosal and subserosal, each with less than half the diameter in the endometrial and peritoneal cavities, respectively. (Van den Bosch T et al. *Ultrasound Obstet Gynecol.* 284–98. 2015. Copyright Wiley-VCH Verlag GmbH & Co. KGaA. Reproduced with permission.)

   The typical US appearance of the myoma is a well-defined, rounded lesion surrounded by or adherent to the myometrium with peripheral blood flow at the color Doppler evaluation. The fibroid can be hypo- or hyperechogenic compared to the myometrial echogenicity. In most cases, shadows are present from the edge of the lesion or linear internal shadows (Figure 6.2).[8] The US aspect of a myoma is related to the amount of muscle cells and fibrous

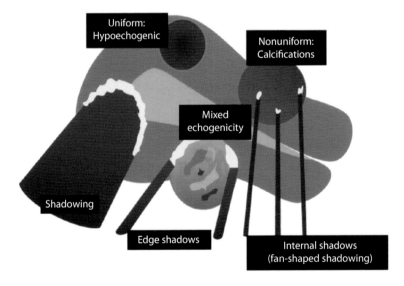

FIGURE 6.2   Ultrasonographic findings of myomas. (Van den Bosch T et al. *Ultrasound Obstet Gynecol.* 284–98. 2015. Copyright Wiley-VCH Verlag GmbH & Co. KGaA. Reproduced with permission.)

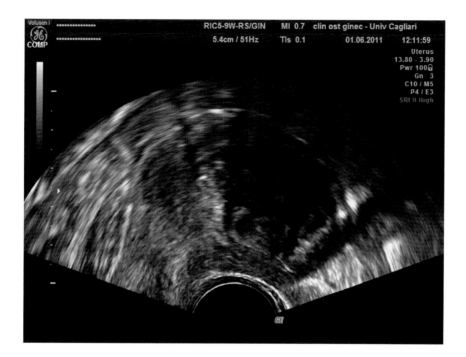

FIGURE 6.3   Intramural myoma.

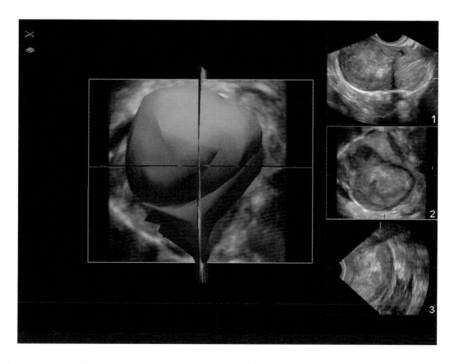

FIGURE 6.4   Three-dimensional ultrasonography rendering of a uterine myoma.

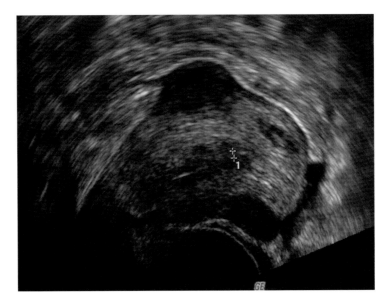

FIGURE 6.5   Subserosal myoma with large base and intramural partially subserous myoma.

stroma present.[9] To correctly program therapeutic options, it is important to evaluate and report for each lesion based on the Morphological Uterus Sonographic Assessment (MUSA)[9] protocol: precise myoma localization (Figures 6.3 through 6.5), dimensions, and US appearance at transvaginal and/or transabdominal scans. Three-dimensional US using 3D multiplanar view (Figures 6.6 and 6.7) of the uterus offers excellent definition of the uterine cavity and the junctional zone (JZ) that are altered by some types of myomas (Figure 6.8).[12]

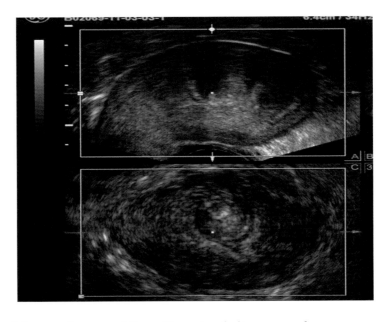

FIGURE 6.6   Submucosal myoma at three-dimensional ultrasonography.

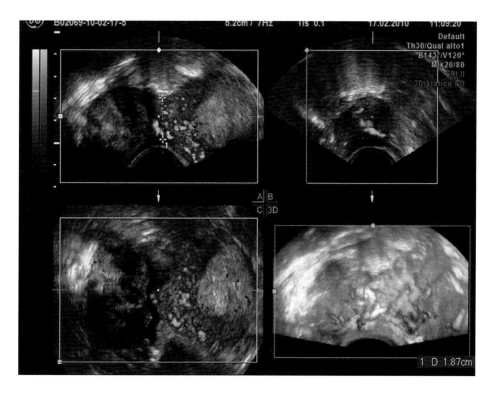

FIGURE 6.7   Infraligament myoma at three-dimensional ultrasonography.

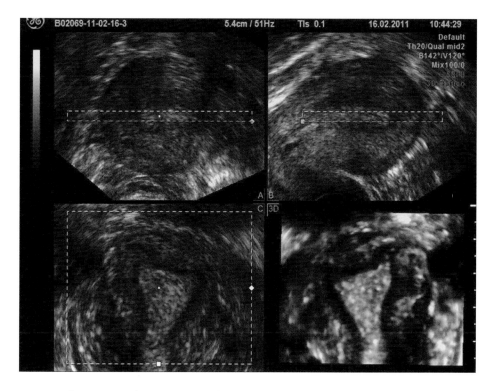

FIGURE 6.8   The junctional zone at three-dimensional coronal plane.

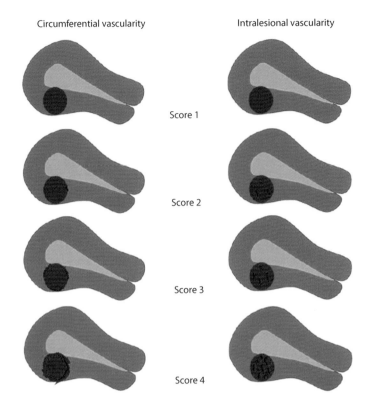

FIGURE 6.9 Vascularization of myomas based on MUSA protocol. (Van den Bosch T et al. *Ultrasound Obstet Gynecol.* 284–98. 2015. Copyright Wiley-VCH Verlag GmbH & Co. KGaA. Reproduced with permission.)

Based on MUSA consensus,[9] if an ill-defined myoma is present, we can subjectively assess the percentage of the whole myometrial volume involved: If it is <50%, the lesion is considered as *localized,* if it is ≥50% of the whole myometrium, it is defined as *global* or *diffuse.*[9]

Using MUSA consensus,[9] we should report vascular assessment of the well-defined myometrial lesions using color and power Doppler techniques.[10–12] The vascular pattern within the myometrium may be described as uniform or nonuniform (Figure 6.9), and the myoma's vascular pattern may be circumferential, intralesional, or both. It is important to note the degrees of vascularization using a subjective color score evaluation of 1, in case of absence of vascularization, to a color score of 4 (Figure 6.10a and b) that refers to abundant color signals. Generally, typical myomas show absent or low internal vascularity (color score 1 or 2) and a well-defined peripheral vascularization (color score 2 or 3) (Figure 6.11a and b).

It is important to differentiate fibroids from adenomyosis (Table 6.1) and malignant degeneration.

ADENOMYOSIS

Adenomyosis is explained in detail in Chapter 5. This disease is due to the extension of endometrial glands and stroma from the endometrium into the myometrium, with an

(a)
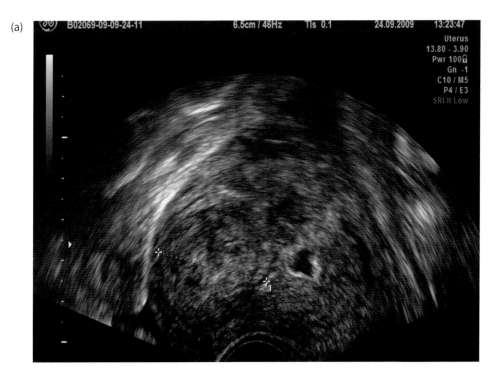

(b)
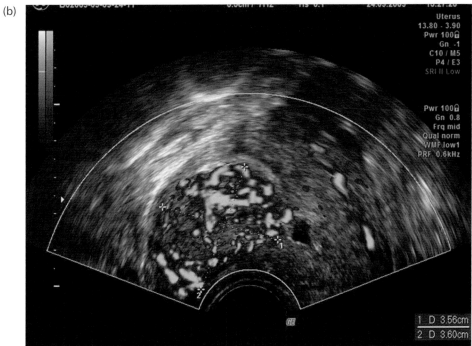

FIGURE 6.10　Myoma with intense vascularization: (a) without and (b) with color Doppler.

(a)

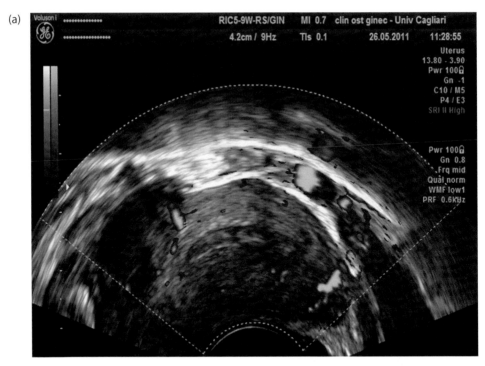

(b)

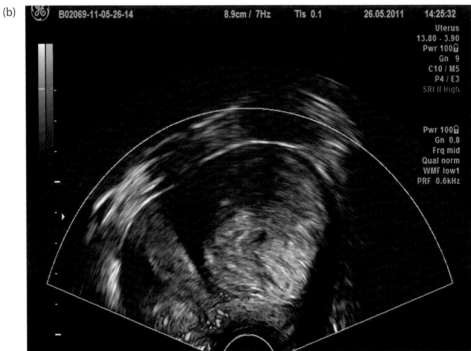

FIGURE 6.11   Typical vascularization of myomas.

TABLE 6.1 Scheme of US Differential Diagnosis between Myoma and Adenomyoma

Myoma	Adenomyoma
Mass that frequently deforms uterine profile	Globular appearance with asymmetry of walls
Presence of pseudocapsule	Undefined margins
Hyperechoic areas (calcifications)	Little anechoic cystic formations
Posterior shadow	Multiple small "comb" shadow cones
Doppler: Prevents peripheral vascularization	Doppler: Not modified vascular structure or widespread hypervascularization

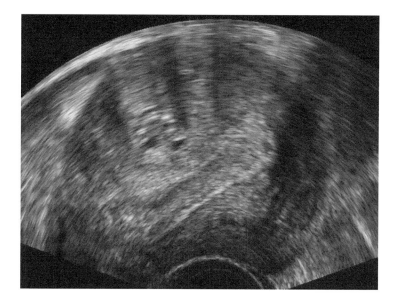

FIGURE 6.12   Small anechoic cysts in the case of adenomyosis.

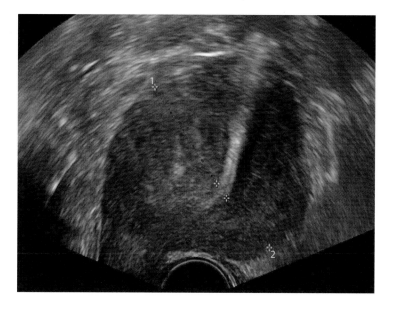

FIGURE 6.13   Asymmetrical thickening in the case of adenomyosis.

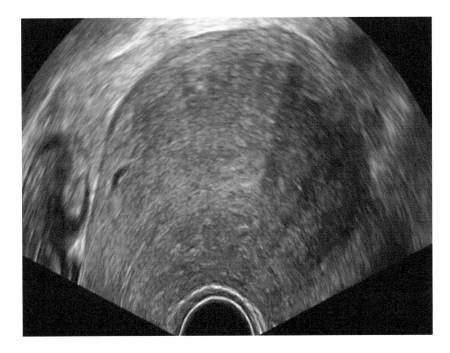

FIGURE 6.14   Fan-shaped shadowing in the case of adenomyosis.

associated growth of the uterus.[13] This gynecological disease is associated with subfertility and pelvic endometriosis.[14,15] Risk factors for adenomyosis are pregnancy termination and cesarean delivery, hormonal (mainly estrogen) exposure, and parity.[16] The clinical presentation may include AUB (menorrhagia), severe dysmenorrhea, and pelvic pain.[17] The US diagnostic features of adenomyosis are a poorly defined JZ, myometrial anechoic cysts or heterogeneous areas (Figure 6.12), asymmetry of the myometrial wall (Figure 6.13), the presence of myometrial hypoechoic linear striations (Figure 6.14), and diffuse vascularity (Figure 6.15a and b).[16,17]

UTERINE SARCOMAS

Uterine sarcomas are malignant uterine tumors that grow from the smooth muscle or connective uterine tissue cells. They represent about 3% of all malignant uterine tumors (Figures 6.16 and 6.17). There are different histological types of sarcoma: leiomyosarcomas and endometrial stromal sarcomas. Leiomyosarcoma (LMS) is the most common sarcoma subtype, which is prevalent among women between the fourth and sixth decade of age. It is generally a single, large myometrial lesion, which causes AUB (56%), a pelvic mass (54%), and pelvic pain (22%).[18] The early symptomatology is very similar to that caused by fibroids, and for this reason, preoperative differential diagnosis is fundamental but may also be difficult. Diagnosis of leiomyosarcoma is histological. Smooth muscle tumors of uncertain malignant potential (STUMPs) are typically solitary uterine tumors, with a large diameter (about 8 cm).[19,20] The US appearance may be similar to fibroids or they may show themselves as heterogeneous masses with necrosis and cystic areas, with irregular vascularization. Frequently, they have an increase of central and circumferential vascularization.

(a)

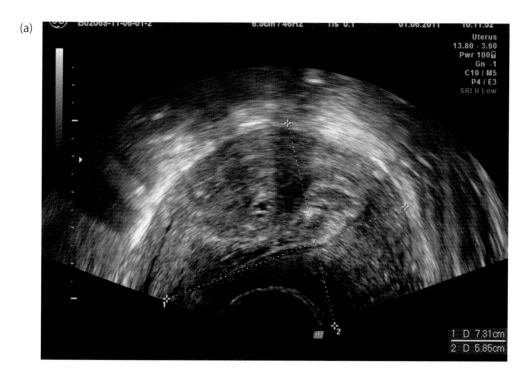

(b)

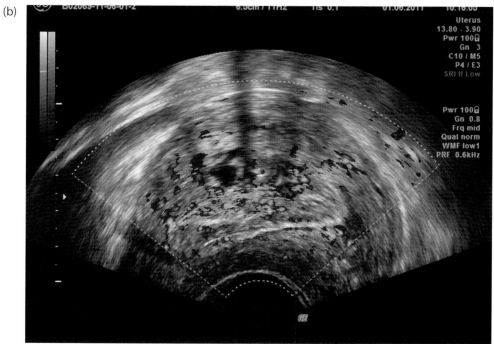

FIGURE 6.15 Translesional vascularization in case of adenomyosis: (a) without and (b) with color Doppler.

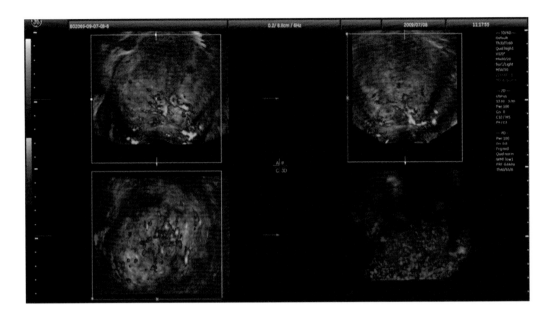

FIGURE 6.16   Ultrasonographic findings of a uterine sarcoma.

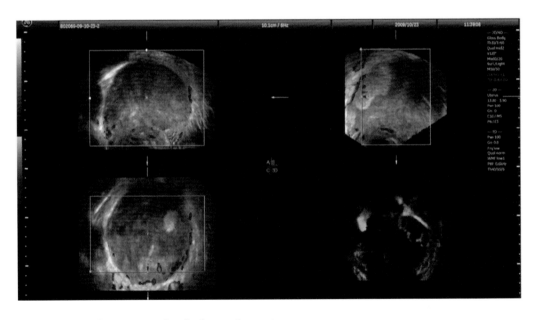

FIGURE 6.17   Ultrasonographic findings of a uterine sarcoma.

REFERENCES

1. Donnez J, Dolmans MM. Uterine fibroid management: From the present to the future. *Hum Reprod Update*. 2016;22:665–86.
2. Singh SS, Belland L, Leyland N, von Riedemann S, Murji A. The past, present, and future of selective progesterone receptor modulators in the management of uterine fibroids. *Am J Obstet Gynecol*. 2018;218:563–572.e1.

3. Tanos V, Berry KE. Benign and malignant pathology of the uterus. *Best Pract Res Clin Obstet Gynecol.* 2018;46:12–30.

4. Simms-Stewart D, Fletcher H. Counselling patients with uterine fibroids: A review of the management and complications. *Obstetrics Gynecol Int.* 2012;2012:1–6.

5. Gupta S, Manyonda IT. Acute complications of fibroids. *Best Pract Res Clin Obstet Gynaecol.* 2009;23:609–17.

6. Rosen M, Anderson M, Hawkins S. Pyomyoma after uterine artery embolization. *Obstetrics Gynecol.* 2013;122:431–3.

7. Kunz G, Beil D, Huppert P, Leyendecker G. Structural abnormalities of the uterine wall in women with endometriosis and infertility visualized by vaginal sonography and magnetic resonance imaging. *Hum Reprod.* 2000;15:76–82.

8. Van den Bosch T. "Adenomyosis and fibroid." *Managing Ultrasonography in Human Reproduction.* Guerriero S et al. (ed). Springer. 2017.

9. Van den Bosch T, Dueholm M, Leone FPG et al. Terms, definitions and measurements to describe sonographic features of myometrium and uterine masses: A consensus opinion from the Morphological Uterus Sonographic Assessment (MUSA) group. *Ultrasound Obstet Gynecol.* 2015;46:284–98.

10. McLucas B. Diagnosis, imaging and anatomical classification of uterine fibroids. *Best Pract Res Clin Obstetrics Gynaecol.* 2008;22:627–42.

11. Dueholm M, Lundorf E, Hansen E, Ledertoug S, Olesen F. Accuracy of magnetic resonance imaging and transvaginal ultrasonography in the diagnosis, mapping, and measurement of uterine myomas. *Am J Obstetrics Gynecol.* 2002;186(3):409–15.

12. Fascilla F, Cramarossa P, Cannone R, Olivieri C, Vimercati A, Exacoustos C. Ultrasound diagnosis of uterine fibroids. *Minerva Ginecol.* 2016;68:297–312.

13. Benagiano G, Habiba M, Brosens I. The pathophysiology of uterine adenomyosis: An update. *Fertil Steril.* 2012;98:572–9.

14. Kissler S, Zangos S, Kohl J, Wiegratz I, Rody A, Gätje R, Vogl TJ, Kunz G, Leyendecker G, Kaufmann M. Duration of dysmenorrhoea and extent of adenomyosis visualised by magnetic resonance imaging. *Eur J Obstetrics Gynecol Reproductive Biol.* 2008;137:204–9.

15. Leyendecker G, Wildt L, Mall G. The pathophysiology of endometriosis and adenomyosis: Tissue injury and repair. *Archives Gynecol Obstetrics.* 2009;280:529–38.

16. Abbott J. Adenomyosis and abnormal uterine bleeding (AUB-A): Pathogenesis, diagnosis, and management. *Best Pract Res Clin Obstetrics Gynaecol.* 2017;40:68–81.

17. Struble J, Reid S, Bedaiwy M. Adenomyosis: A clinical review of a challenging gynecologic condition. *J Minim Invasive Gynecol.* 2016;23:164–85.

18. Khan A, Shehmar M, Gupta J. Uterine fibroids: Current perspectives. *Int J Women's Health.* 2014;6:95–114.

19. Exacoustos C, Romanini M, Amadio A, Amoroso C, Szabolcs B, Zupi E, Arduini D. Can gray-scale and color Doppler sonography differentiate between uterine leiomyosarcoma and leiomyoma? *J Clin Ultrasound.* 2007;35:449–57.

20. Valentin L. Imaging techniques in the management of abnormal vaginal bleeding in non-pregnant women before and after menopause. *Best Pract Res Clin Obstetrics Gynaecol.* 2014;28:637–54.

21. Munro MG, Critchley HO, Broder MS, Fraser IS. FIGO classification system (PALM-COEIN) for causes of abnormal uterine bleeding in nongravid women of reproductive age. *Int J Gynaecol Obstet.* 2011;113(1):3–13.

CHAPTER 7

Müllerian Anomalies

Betlem Graupera and Jean L. Browne

INTRODUCTION

Müllerian anomalies are a heterogeneous group of congenital anomalies caused by isolated or complex alterations happening at different stages of embryological development, whether in the formation, channeling, fusion, or absorption of the Müllerian ducts. They can occur as single defects or as a combination of defects, the latter resulting in so-called complex anomalies.[1–3]

The prevalence of these malformations is variable and mainly related to the cohort studied, reported in about 5.5% of the general population and in up to 24.5% of infertile patients with a history of miscarriage.[4]

There are different classifications for uterine malformations. The most used classification was that of the American Fertility Society (AFS) of 1988.[5] However, the European Society of Human Reproduction and Embryology and the European Society for Gynecological Endoscopy (ESHRE-ESGE) recently published a new consensus on the classification of congenital malformations of the female genital tract.[2]

There are several techniques for the diagnosis of uterine malformations. Many authors have shown that conventional ultrasound is a useful technique for the evaluation of Müllerian malformations.[6–9] Although two-dimensional ultrasound (2DUS) can easily identify some anomalies, such as a bicornuate uterus, it has serious limitations to identify other types of malformations, such as a hemi-uterus.[10] Pascual et al. demonstrated that a uterine transverse diameter less than 45 mm could significantly exclude a canalization defect.[11] Three-dimensional ultrasound (3DUS) has been shown to be very accurate in the diagnosis of uterine malformations.[12]

Women with Müllerian anomalies can be asymptomatic[13] or can present with gynecological symptoms, including pelvic pain and/or presence of a mass due to obstruction of the outflow of menstrual residue with hematocolpos and hematometra, as well as infertility and miscarriage.[14] Noteworthy are the obstetric complications: spontaneous abortion, preterm delivery, malpresentation at delivery, low birth weight, and perinatal mortality. These happen at higher rates in pregnant women with Müllerian anomalies than in pregnant women without Müllerian anomalies.[15] Congenital uterine anomalies may be associated with other congenital anomalies, which most frequently are anomalies of the urinary tract.[16]

In this chapter we will review the ultrasonographic findings of uterine anomalies with emphasis on those related to pelvic pain.

CLASSIFICATION OF MÜLLERIAN ANOMALIES

The ESHRE-ESGE classification is based on the degree of anatomical distortion, beginning with the least severe (Class U1) to the most extreme (Class U5). The normal uterus is classified as U0, whereas those that are deemed not classifiable are in Class U6.

Class U0: Normal Uterus

The normal uterus viewed on a two-dimensional ultrasound has a "pear-shaped" morphology on sagittal sections. The external contour of the corpus is convex, with no concavities seen on any plane. The endometrium reflects as a central bright echogenic line on all planes. Cephalic cross sections of the corpus show this bright line in a central position extending toward the uterine horns.

Coronal reconstructions of 3DUS show a slightly convex outer contour. A coronal view also reveals the triangular shape of the endometrium with a flat or slightly concave or convex silhouette at the fundal level (Figure 7.1).

Class U1: Dysmorphic Uterus

According to the ESHRE-ESGE consensus, Class U1 includes all uteri with a normal outer uterine contour but with an abnormal uterine cavity shape, excluding septa. Class U1 is divided in three categories: Class U1a or T-shaped uterus; Class U1b or uterus infantilis; and finally Class U1c, which includes minor deformities of the uterine cavity.[2]

Two-dimensional ultrasound findings of a class U1a dysmorphic uterus are unspecific but may be suspected in any patient with a small uterus.

A three-dimensional coronal reveals a narrow instead of widening triangular morphology of the endometrium resulting in its typical tubular "T" morphology (Figure 7.2).

Class U2: Septate Uterus

A septate uterus occurs due a failure in the resorption of the septum resulting from the medial fusion of both Müllerian ducts. There are two subclasses: partial septum or Class U2a, and complete septum or Class U2b.[2]

The outer contour of a septate uterus on 2DUS is of convex shape, although it may be flat or slightly concave. The endometrium is divided in two refringent areas separated by a layer of myometrial tissue, which represents the uterine septum (Figure 7.3). The septum tissue can reach the cervix and is therefore called a complete septum, or it can end at any point of the uterine cavity in the partial septum, with a single endometrial line at lower sections.

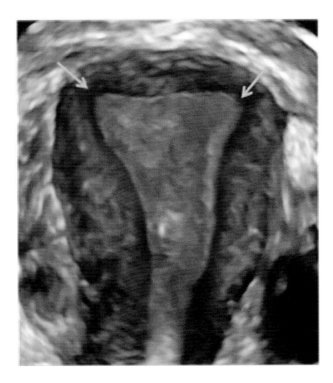

FIGURE 7.1 Three-dimensional ultrasound coronal image of a normal uterus clearly shows the normal external contour at the fundal level of the uterus and the normal triangular shape of the endometrial cavity with the interstitial portion of both fallopian tubes as reference points (arrows).

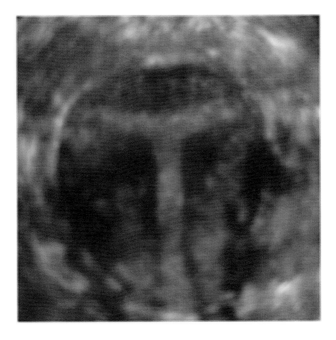

FIGURE 7.2 Three-dimensional rendered coronal view of a dysmorphic uterus (Class U1a) demonstrating the T-shape morphology of the uterine cavity.

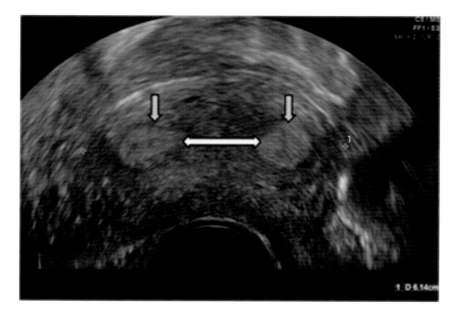

FIGURE 7.3   Two-dimensional ultrasound cross section of a septate uterus shows an enlarged uterine transverse diameter. The higher cross section level shows two refringent areas corresponding to the endometrium (yellow arrows) and separated by myometrial tissue corresponding to the uterine septum (double white arrow).

Three-dimensional ultrasound shows a normal external contour. Two refringent areas corresponding to the endometrium are separated by a myometrial septum borne from the fundal midline; its length exceeds 50% of the uterine wall thickness. This myometrial tissue can protrude in the uterine cavity without reaching the internal cervical os, therefore a partial septum (Figure 7.4), or extend through the entire uterine cavity up to the level of the internal cervical os, the complete septate uterus. The lower part of the septum may appear more hypoechogenic due to its more fibrous nature (Figure 7.5).

Class U3: Bicorporeal Uterus

Anomalies resulting from a lack of both partial and total fusion of the Müllerian ducts are included in a single group in the ESHRE-ESGE consensus: Class U3 or bicorporal uterus. This class is further divided in three subclasses: Class U3a or partial bicorporal uterus, Class U3b or complete bicorporal uterus, and Class U3c or bicorporal septate uterus.[2] The complete bicorporal uterus is known as didelphys uterus in the AFS classification.[5]

Two-dimensional ultrasound cross sections demonstrate an external myometrial contour indentation between the two uterine horns. Two echogenic zones corresponding to the endometrium, one in each horn, are also seen. These two endometrial images can be followed from the fundus to the internal cervical os or can be interrupted at any point of the uterine cavity, with a single endometrial line reaching the cervix, reflecting whether it is a complete, septate, or partial bicorporeal uterus.

Three-dimensional ultrasound of a bicorporal uterus reveals two divergent and symmetrical uterine horns; a deep cleft on its outer contour, greater than 50% of the uterine

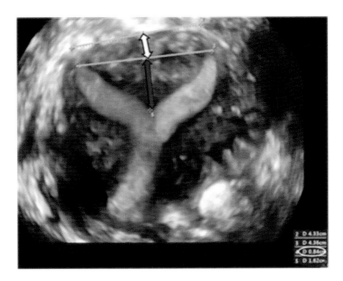

FIGURE 7.4 Three-dimensional ultrasound rendered image of a partial septate uterus showing a slightly convex external uterine contour and a septum partially dividing the uterine cavity. This figure illustrates myometrial wall thickness measurement (double white arrow). Thickness is measured at the fundal level in a coronal view from the external contour to the interostial line (yellow line). In this case, the length of the septum (double red arrow) exceeds 50% of the uterine wall thickness.

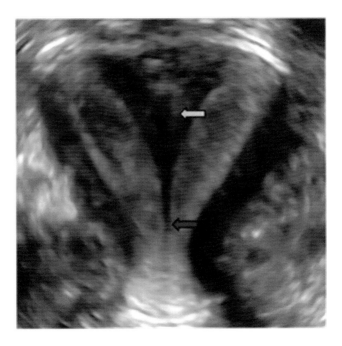

FIGURE 7.5 Three-dimensional ultrasound rendered image of a complete septate uterus showing a slightly convex external uterine contour and a septum completely dividing the uterine cavity (yellow arrow). Note that the lower part of the septum appears more hypoechogenic due to its more fibrous nature (red arrow).

wall thickness, ends above the level of the cervix in a partial bicorporal uterus (U3a) (Figure 7.6) or reaches the level of the cervix in a complete bicorporal uterus (U3b) (Figure 7.7). The bicorporal septate uterus (U3c) is characterized by the presence of an absorption defect in addition to the main fusion defect (Figure 7.8). In these cases, 3DUS shows that the deepness of the midline fundal cleft is more than 150% of the uterine wall thickness.

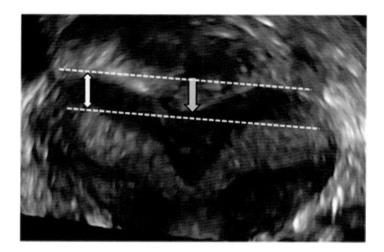

FIGURE 7.6 Three-dimensional ultrasound rendered image of a partial bicorporeal uterus, demonstrating the two uterine horns separated by an external cleft (yellow arrow) deeper than 50% of the uterine wall thickness (white arrow). This image demonstrates the cavity partially divided above the level of the cervix.

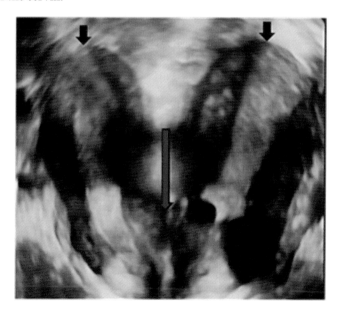

FIGURE 7.7 Three-dimensional ultrasound rendered image of a complete bicorporeal uterus, demonstrating two separate uterine horns (black arrows) and an external cleft separating both horns that reaches the level of the cervix (red arrow).

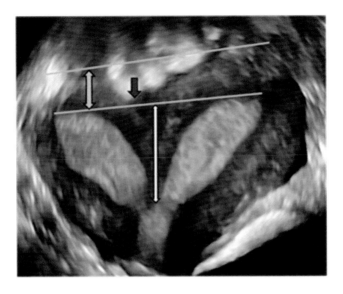

FIGURE 7.8   Three-dimensional ultrasound rendered image of a bicorporeal septate uterus, showing the external cleft (red arrow) between both uterine horns and a septum dividing the uterine cavity (white arrow), exceeding by 50% the uterine wall thickness (double yellow arrow).

Class U4: Hemi-Uterus

The hemi-uterus, the unicornuate in the AFS classification,[5] results from the development of a single Müllerian duct, while the contralateral duct could be either incompletely formed or absent.

In the ESHRE-ESGE consensus, this unilateral formation defect is divided in two subclasses depending on the presence or absence of a functional endometrium in the rudimentary horn. Class U4a, or hemi-uterus with a rudimentary cavity, is defined by the presence of a normal hemi-uterus with a communicating or noncommunicating functional endometrium in a rudimentary contralateral horn. Class U4b, or hemi-uterus without a rudimentary cavity, is characterized either by the presence of a rudimentary horn without a functional endometrium or by aplasia of the contralateral part.

The ultrasound findings observed by 2DUS in this class of anomalies are subtle. It may be suggested by a reduced transverse diameter of the uterus that is lateralized toward an adnexal region in the pelvis. The refringent image corresponding to the endometrium may appear eccentric inside the myometrium in the transverse sections. A methodical exploration of the pelvis to identify a rudimentary horn is mandatory; it can be seen as a much smaller hemi-uterus (Figure 7.9).

Using 3DUS the hemi-uterus appears curved and elongated, presenting the banana external morphology that has been previously described by magnetic resonance imaging. The uterine volume is reduced, and the configuration of the uterus is asymmetric. The endometrium may be uniformly narrow or may be bullet shaped, tapering at the apex (Figure 7.10).[17] Three-dimensional ultrasound might reveal whether a rudimentary horn is present. The nonfunctional rudimentary horn is usually much smaller than the functional rudimentary horn, thus making accurate diagnosis more difficult. It is important to

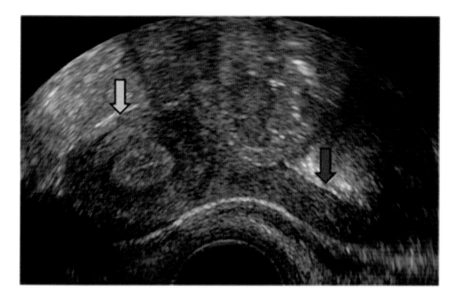

FIGURE 7.9   Two-dimensional ultrasound showing a uterine cross section deviated to the right side, corresponding to a hemi-uterus (yellow arrow). On the left side there is a mass with the same echogenicity as the uterus, which corresponds to a rudimentary horn without functional endometrium (red arrow).

consider the differential diagnosis between a rudimentary horn and a pelvic mass, such as a myoma or an adnexal mass.

Class U5: Hypoplasia and Agenesis

The Class U5 group of uterine anomalies results from the incomplete development of one or both Müllerian ducts, mainly represented by a small uterus. Women with these anomalies have uterine remnants without endometrial cavities and/or unilateral or bilateral rudimentary horns with small endometrial cavities.

Class U5 is further divided into two subclasses: Class U5a, or aplastic uterus with a rudimentary cavity, which is characterized by the presence of endometrium in either one or both horns; and Class U5b, or aplastic uterus without a rudimentary cavity, when there is either presence of uterine remnants or full uterine agenesis.[2]

The ultrasound findings reflect the grade of anomaly. In cases of uterine agenesis, no uterine images are detected. In these cases, the cervix and vagina may also not be seen. If there is a uterine remnant, ultrasound will reveal a very small uterine image that might have a functional endometrial cavity (Figure 7.11). If there is no vagina, a transabdominal ultrasound should be performed (Figure 7.12).

Cervical Anomalies

According to the ESHRE-ESGE consensus, cervical morphology is divided in five subclasses. Subclass C0, or normal cervix, incorporates all forms of normal cervical development. Subclass C1, or septate, is defined by a cervical resorption defect with a normal external cervix and a septum dividing the cervical canal. Subclass C2, or double cervix, incorporates

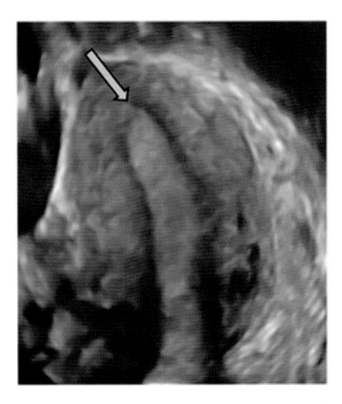

FIGURE 7.10   Three-dimensional ultrasound rendered image shows the external banana morphology and the abnormal lenticular shape of the uterine cavity pertaining to a single right horn (yellow arrow).

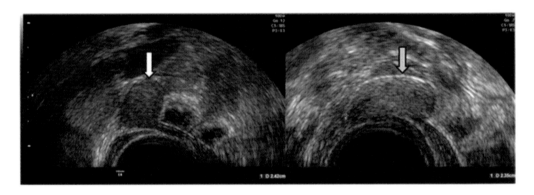

FIGURE 7.11   Two-dimensional ultrasound shows two uterine remnants. The right uterine remnant is 24 mm (white arrow) and the left uterine remnant is 23 mm (yellow arrow).

all cases of complete cervical fusion defects and is defined by two distinct externally rounded cervices that can be either fully distinct or partially fused. Subclass C3, or unilateral cervical aplasia, is defined by the unilateral development of one cervix. Subclass C4, or cervical aplasia, incorporates all cases of complete cervical aplasia as well as those with severe cervical formation defects.[2] Bermejo et al. considered the presence of two diverging cervical canals on 3DUS as criteria to diagnose two cervices. Ultrasonographic study of the cervix improves

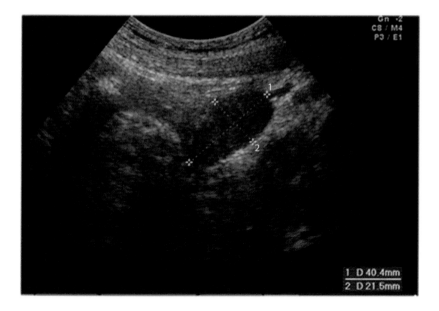

FIGURE 7.12   Transabdominal ultrasound shows a uterine remnant without functional endometrium and vaginal agenesis in a patient afflicted with Mayer-Rokitansky-Küster-Hauser syndrome.

during the periovulatory phase of the menstrual cycle, because the endocervical mucus in this phase enhances visualization of the cervical canal (Figures 7.13 through 7.15).[18]

Vaginal Anomalies

The ESHRE-ESGE consensus also provides a five-subclass classification that describes the normal vagina and its anomalies: Subclass V0, or normal vagina, incorporates all cases of normal vaginal development (Figure 7.16); Subclass V1, with a longitudinal nonobstructing vaginal septum; Subclass V2, with a longitudinal obstructing vaginal septum; Subclass V3, with a transverse vaginal septum and/or imperforate hymen; and Subclass V4, or vaginal aplasia, incorporates all cases of complete or partial vaginal aplasia.[2]

The introduction of gel in the vagina improves its study as described by Bermejo et al., allowing visualization of the vaginal anatomy from the transperineal 3DUS volume (Figures 7.17 and 7.18).[19]

PELVIC PAIN AND MÜLLERIAN ANOMALIES

Müllerian Anomalies and Endometriosis

There are many causes of pelvic pain. One of the most common causes of pelvic pain is due to the presence of endometriosis. Women with uterine anomalies may also present with pelvic pain caused by adenomyosis (Figure 7.19).

The most widely accepted theory as to the etiology of endometriosis was proposed by Sampson in 1927.[20] According to the theory of retrograde menstruation, endometriosis may be due to the existence of Müllerian anomalies causing obstruction of the menstruation outflow tract, such as complete transverse vaginal septum, imperforate hymen, and cervical agenesis.[21,22]

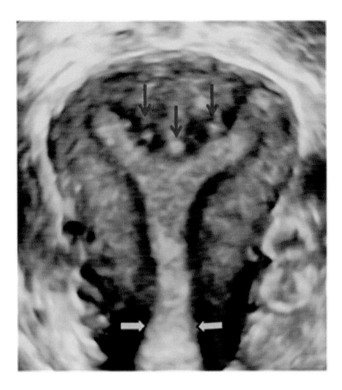

FIGURE 7.13   Three-dimensional ultrasound rendered image showing a coronal view of a partial septate uterus with one single cervix. The yellow arrows are pointing to the single cervix. Note the presence of subendometrial buds (red arrows) characteristic of adenomyosis.

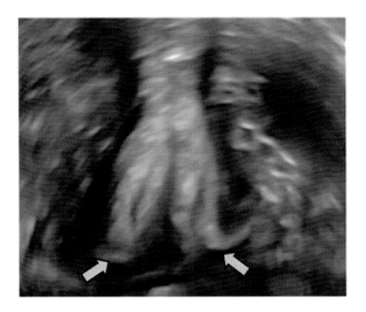

FIGURE 7.14   Three-dimensional ultrasound coronal view of a double cervix. The arrows are pointing to two divergent cervical canals.

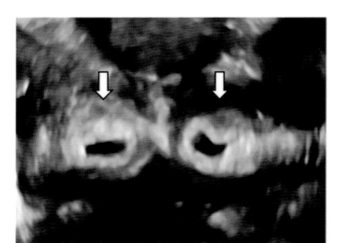

FIGURE 7.15   Three-dimensional transvaginal ultrasound rendered image of the cervix of a woman with double cervix. The transverse plane at the level of the external cervical os shows the two external cervical openings (arrows).

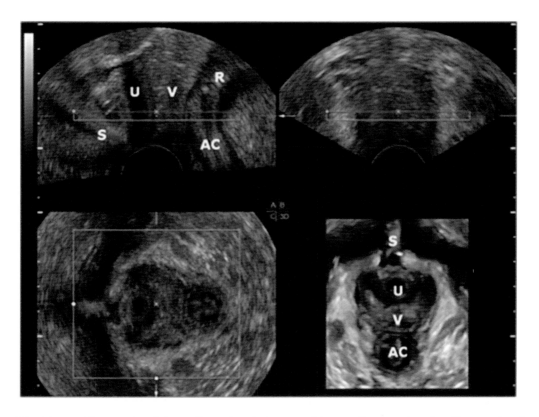

FIGURE 7.16   Transperineal three-dimensional ultrasound image of a normal vagina. Transperineal acquisition of the pelvic floor is done in a sagittal plane (Window A), identifying, from anterior to posterior, the pubic symphysis (S), urethra (U), vagina (V), rectum (R), and anal canal (AC). The rendered image (3D) clearly shows the normal vagina.

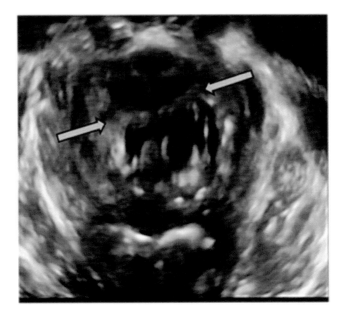

FIGURE 7.17 Transperineal three-dimensional ultrasound image shows a vagina with a septum dividing it (arrows). The vagina has been filled with gel to improve its imaging.

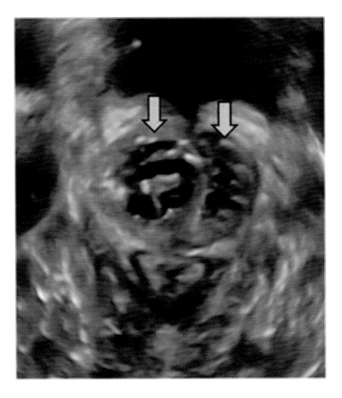

FIGURE 7.18 Transperineal three-dimensional ultrasound view of a double vagina in a woman with a bicorporal septate uterus and double cervix. Both hemivaginas have been filled with gel. Arrows are pointing to both hemivaginas.

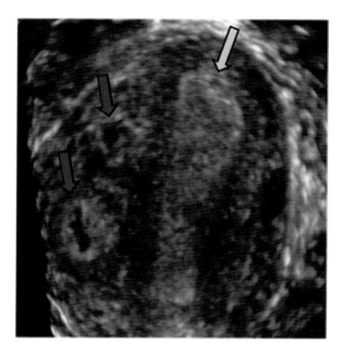

FIGURE 7.19 Three-dimensional ultrasound rendered image shows a hemi-uterus with adenomyosis. Notice the abnormal banana shape of the hemi-uterus with the bullet shape of the uterine cavity (yellow arrow). Notice also round cystic images within the myometrium, characteristic of adenomyosis (red arrows).

Other investigators such as, Nawroth et al., observed that endometriosis has also been associated with nonobstructive Müllerian anomalies.[23] LaMonica et al. observed that the presence of a uterine septum as well as other factors may predispose women endometriosis, especially for stage IV of the disease.[24] Previously, Leyendecker et al. had demonstrated uterine dysperistalsis as a mechanism for the development of endometriosis.[25] Nawroth et al. suggested that a septate uterus may contribute to this disturbed peristalsis, enabling retrograde menstruation, and therefore an increased risk of developing endometriosis.[23] Matalliotakis et al. found that adolescent young girls with endometriosis had uterine malformations to a greater extent than the group without endometriosis. They reported that the septate uterus is the most obvious type of Müllerian defect associated with endometriosis.[26]

Obstructive Anomalies

According to Zhang et al., obstructive anomalies of the female genital tract in patients who present with primary amenorrhea and cyclical pelvic pain, include transverse vaginal septum, imperforate hymen, cervical anomalies, and a hemi-uterus with a noncommunicating functional rudimentary horn.[27]

There are other anomalies, which are associated with pelvic pain due to obstruction of the menstrual outflow, including the presence of a longitudinal vaginal septum in the context of Wünderlich syndrome and cervical agenesis associated with complete bicornuate uterus. Mayer-Rokitansky-Küster-Hauser syndrome and Robert's uterus are also related to pelvic pain.

Transverse Vaginal Septum

The transverse vaginal septum is a rare malformation that affects approximately 1/80,000 newborns. It seems to be due to a failure in the fusion or channeling of the urogenital sinus and the Müllerian ducts. It is usually observed in the upper and middle third of the vagina. It is rarely associated with uterine malformations.

Women with transverse vaginal septum have hematocolpos due to obstruction of the menstrual outflow if the septum is not perforated. Pyohematocolpos, although rare, may develop if ascending infection occurs in the case of a microperforated septum. These women also present with dyspareunia.[28]

Imperforate Hymen

The main anomaly of the hymen is complete closure. The prevalence is 0.1% and usually appears as an isolated finding. The imperforate hymen represents a failure in the final process of canalization of the vagina with similar clinical and imaging findings as those of the transverse vaginal septum (Figure 7.20).[29]

Longitudinal Vaginal Septum

The longitudinal vaginal septum represents failure of the complete canalization of the vagina. It is frequently associated with congenital uterine anomalies.[30] An obstructed hemivagina results when the caudal longitudinal vaginal septum attaches to the internal vaginal wall. The presence of this septum prevents menstruation outflow.[31] Patients affected with this septum present with cyclical pelvic pain due to the presence of hematocolpos and/or hematometra (Figure 7.17).

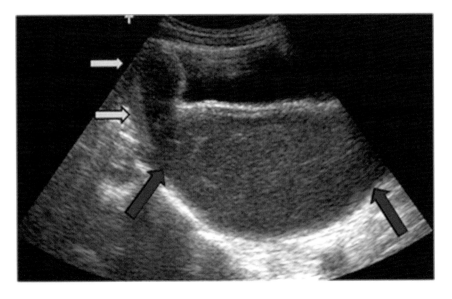

FIGURE 7.20   Transabdominal ultrasound in a pubescent girl shows the presence of hematocolpos (red arrows) and hematometra (yellow arrows) due to obstruction of the menstrual outflow caused by an imperforate hymen.

Cervical Anomalies

Cervical anomalies can be classified according to the ESHRE-ESGE classification.[2] Patients with cervical agenesis and with a functioning endometrium present with primary amenorrhea and cyclic pelvic pain due to the obstruction to menstrual outflow. The presence of a normal uterus and an abnormal cervix is infrequent. Patients with cervical anomalies have vaginal agenesis in 50% of cases, particularly those with cervical agenesis. One-third of them will have a uterine anomaly.[32] Xie et al. described four types of cervical atresia. Ultrasound reveals liquid accumulation in the uterine cavity and a variable degree of cervical anomalies (Figure 7.21).[33]

Herlyn-Werner-Wünderlich Syndrome

The Herlyn-Werner-Wünderlich syndrome was initially described by Purslow.[34] It is a complex anomaly that includes uterus didelphys, obstructed hemivagina, and ipsilateral renal agenesis. This syndrome, also known as Wünderlich syndrome and OHVIRA (obstructed hemivagina and ipsilateral renal anomaly), is an unsuspected diagnosis entity since the patient presents normal menstrual flow from the unobstructed hemi-uterus.[35] Although classically this syndrome has been reported in the didelphys uterus, it has also been observed in the complete septate uterus (Figures 7.22 through 7.25).[36]

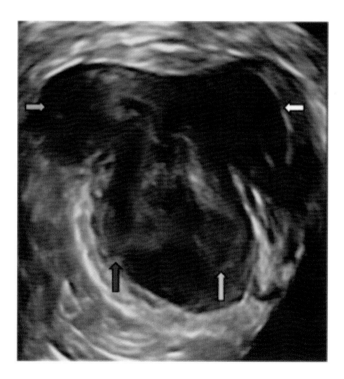

FIGURE 7.21   Three-dimensional ultrasound rendered image of a bicorporeal uterus, demonstrating two separate uterine horns (right horn: blue arrow; left horn: white arrow) and two cervical canals. The right cervical canal shows a normal external cervical os (red arrow), while the left cervical canal shows a stop at the lower third (yellow arrow) and no external cervical opening is detected. The left uterine horn shows liquid accumulation in the uterine cavity due to the left cervical anomaly.

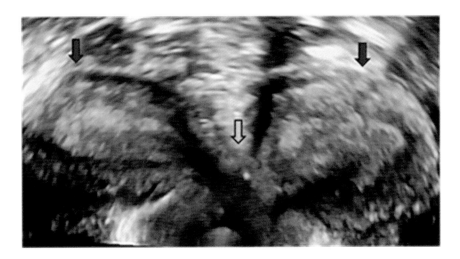

FIGURE 7.22 Woman afflicted with Wünderlich syndrome (same patient through Figure 7.25). Three-dimensional ultrasound rendered image of a complete bicorporeal uterus, demonstrating two separate uterine horns (red arrows) and an external cleft between the horns that extends to the level of the cervix (yellow arrow).

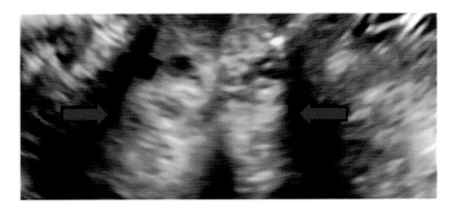

FIGURE 7.23 Woman with Wünderlich syndrome. Three-dimensional ultrasound rendered image showing a coronal view of the cervix. The arrows are pointing to two divergent cervical canals.

Hemi-Uterus with a Rudimentary Cavity

Women who have a hemi-uterus with a noncommunicating functional endometrium in a rudimentary horn present a higher incidence of adenomyosis in the rudimentary horn as well as endometriosis in other locations (Figures 7.26 through 7.29). These patients will present pelvic pain, a pelvic mass, hematometra, hematosalpinx by obstruction of menstrual outflow, and infertility. The clinical symptoms usually manifest at menarche. Other patients may be asymptomatic and only diagnosed when complaining due to infertility.[14,27,37–40]

Hypoplasia and Agenesis: Mayer-Rokitansky-Küster-Hauser Syndrome

Mayer-Rokitansky-Küster-Hauser syndrome is characterized by a variable degree of uterine and vaginal underdevelopment. Women with this syndrome may present aplasia of the

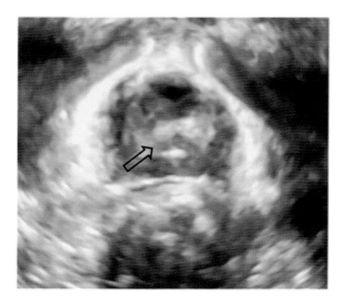

FIGURE 7.24   Woman with Wünderlich syndrome. Transperineal three-dimensional ultrasound image shows a vagina with a dividing septum (arrow).

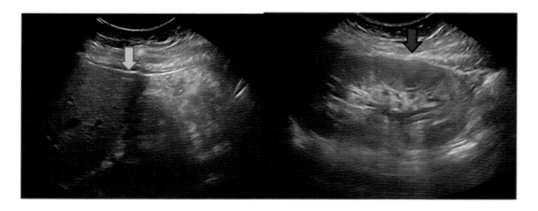

FIGURE 7.25   Woman with Wünderlich syndrome. Two-dimensional ultrasound showing a left kidney alone (red arrow). Note the absence of the right kidney (yellow arrow).

uterus, cervix, and the upper part of the vagina, although they can also exhibit small uterine, cervical, and/or tubal vestiges (Figure 7.12). Abnormalities of the upper urinary tract are present in 30% to 40% of patients with this syndrome.[41] These patients are diagnosed at puberty, presenting with amenorrhea and severe pelvic pain due to hematometra caused by obstructive defects if there is a functional endometrium but vaginal agenesis. The reproductive possibilities depend on the degree of the anomaly, mainly the presence of a functional endometrium.[17] As Hall-Craggs et al. described, a rudimentary uterus is common in Mayer-Rokitansky-Küster-Hauser syndrome.[42] This rudimentary uterus can be relatively large and have a functional endometrium and engender pelvic pain. Wang et al. observed that patients with Mayer-Rokitansky-Küster-Hauser syndrome had a history of cyclic pelvic pain that was more common in women with a unilateral rudimentary uterus compared to

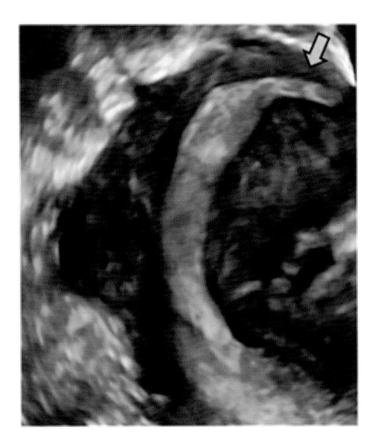

FIGURE 7.26   Three-dimensional ultrasound rendered image shows a banana external morphology and a left endometrial (yellow arrow).

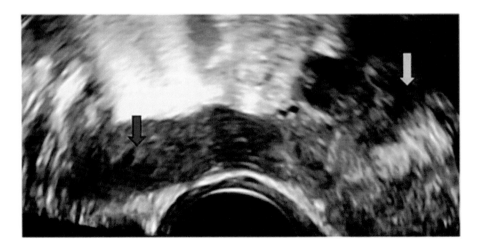

FIGURE 7.27   Hemi-uterus (yellow arrow) (same patient as Figure 7.26). Three-dimensional ultrasound also reveals a noncommunicating rudimentary horn with functional endometrium (red arrow).

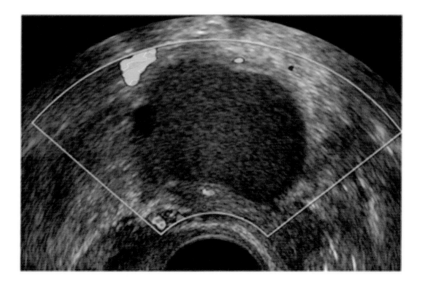

FIGURE 7.28   Woman with hemi-uterus and functional rudimentary horn (same patient as Figures 7.26 and 7.27) who also had an endometriotic ovarian cyst, with characteristic ground-glass pattern.

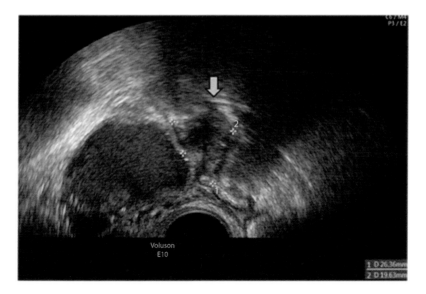

FIGURE 7.29   Two-dimensional ultrasound shows an endometriotic nodule infiltrating the rectum and the left utero-sacral ligament in a woman presenting a hemi-uterus with functional rudimentary horn (same patient as Figures 7.26 through 7.28).

those with no rudimentary uterus or with bilateral uterine remnants.[43] Endometriosis was more frequent in patients with a unilateral rudimentary uterus.

Robert's Uterus

Robert's uterus is a rare congenital Müllerian duct anomaly. It was first described by Robert in 1969.[44] It is characterized by a septate uterus with a noncommunicating hemicavity and a normal external uterine contour.

Patients with Robert's uterus present with recurrent abdominal pain and dysmenorrhea caused by hematometra, hematosalpinx, and in some cases endometriosis as a result of the restriction in the menstrual outflow. These patients can also present with acute pelvic pain.[45] There are few cases reported in the literature.[46] Di Spiezio Sardo et al. describe a case of Robert's uterus as a complete septate uterus with unilateral cervical aplasia (U2bC3V0) using the ESHRE-ESGE classification.[47] The use of three-dimensional ultrasound allows a precise representation of the female genital anatomy even in the presence of complex anomalies as in the case of Robert's uterus.[46,47]

Uterine Anomalies, Pregnancy, and Pelvic Pain

Some pregnant patients with uterine malformations may appear to have an ectopic pregnancy. As a general rule, gynecological and obstetric complications are more frequent in women with uterine anomalies (Figures 7.30 and 7.31).[15,48]

In patients with a hemi-uterus, pregnancy may implant in either one of the two cavities, causing different obstetrical and maternal outcomes. Pregnancy in a noncommunicating rudimentary hemi-uterus is associated with adverse reproductive outcomes such as an increase in miscarriage, preterm labor, and malpresentation.[49] If the pregnancy occurs in the noncommunicating horn, it is considered an ectopic pregnancy. In such cases, the obstetrical outcomes are very poor, with an increased risk of miscarriage, preterm labor, malpresentation, intrauterine growth restriction, intrauterine fetal death, and placenta accrete.[50] Nevertheless, the most life-threatening condition is uterine rupture due to the thin myometrium that is normally found in

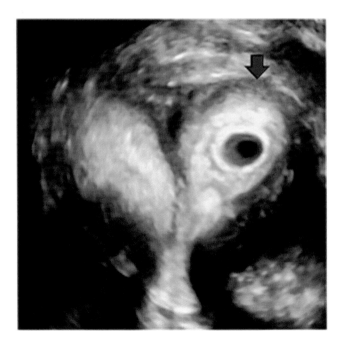

FIGURE 7.30   Three-dimensional ultrasound clearly shows the pregnancy in the left cavity of a septate uterus (red arrow).

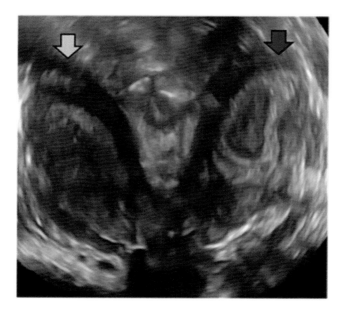

FIGURE 7.31 Three-dimensional ultrasound demonstrates a complete bicorporeal uterus with an empty right horn (yellow arrow) and a pregnancy in the left uterine horn (red arrow).

rudimentary horns, presenting as an acute gynecologic emergency with abdominal pain and severe hemoperitoneum. The incidence of rudimentary horn pregnancy is low, but the rate of rupture is close to 80%.[51]

Ectopic pregnancy in a rudimentary horn has distinctive ultrasonographic features. Tsafrir et al. described a pseudopattern of an asymmetrical bicornuate uterus, with no visual continuity between the cervical canal and the lumen of the pregnant horn, the presence of myometrial tissue enclosing the gestational sac, and, additionally, hypervascularization typical of placenta accrete. Ultrasound reveals a very thin myometrium surrounding the pregnancy, which might be confused with an adnexal gestational sac and the presence of the empty cavity in the larger uterine horn.[52] Three-dimensional ultrasound demonstrates the abnormal lenticular shape of the hemi-uterus and a pregnant contralateral rudimentary horn. Two-dimensional ultrasonographic suspicion and ultrasonographic features confirmed by three-dimensional ultrasound warrant the diagnosis, as suggested by Blancafort et al. (Figures 7.32 and 7.33).[53]

In the presence of uterine malformations, pregnancy should be very carefully managed. Three-dimensional ultrasound provides precise details about the localization of pregnancy in patients presenting with uterine anomalies and pelvic pain, allowing reliable differential diagnosis with an ectopic pregnancy.

SUMMARY

Ultrasound, especially 3DUS, allows a detailed study of the female genital anatomy even in the presence of complex anomalies. Ultrasound is a useful technique to evaluate the female pelvis in patients presenting with uterine abnormalities and pelvic pain, and offers a unique opportunity for treatment planning of these cases.

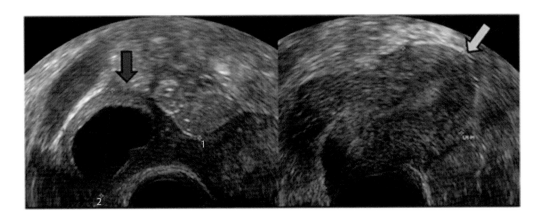

FIGURE 7.32 Two-dimensional ultrasound images show on the left hemi-uterus with its empty uterine cavity (yellow arrow). On the right side a pregnancy in the noncommunicating rudimentary horn (red arrow) can be seen. When there is no pregnancy or endometrium in the rudimentary horn, differential diagnosis of the rudimentary horn with pelvic masses such as a myoma or an adnexal mass should be entertained.

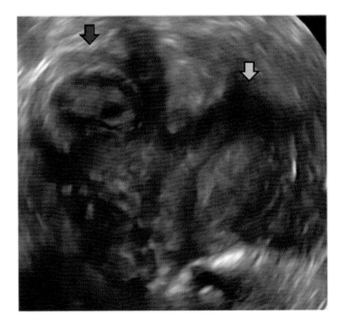

FIGURE 7.33 (Same patient as Figure 7.32.) Three-dimensional ultrasound rendered image showing a coronal uterine view of the left side, corresponding to a hemi-uterus, with its empty uterine cavity (yellow arrow). On the right side a pregnancy in the noncommunicating rudimentary horn can be observed (red arrow).

ACKNOWLEDGMENTS

Under the auspices of the Càtedra d' Investigació en Obstetrícia i Ginecologia de la Universitat Autònoma de Barcelona. Thanks to Beatriz Valero for help in the editing of this work.

REFERENCES

1. Grimbizis GF, Camus M, Tarlatzis BC, Bontis JN, Devroey P. Clinical implications of uterine malformations and hysteroscopic treatment results. *Hum Reprod Update.* 2001;7:161–74.
2. Grimbizis GF, Gordts S, Di Spiezio Sardo A et al. The ESHRE/ESGE consensus on the classification of female genital tract congenital anomalies. *Hum Reprod.* 2013;28:2032–44.
3. Grimbizis GF, Di Spiezio Sardo A, Saravelos SH et al. The Thessaloniki ESHRE/ESGE consensus on diagnosis of female genital anomalies. *Gynecol Surg.* 2016;13:1–16.
4. Chan YY, Jayaprakasan K, Zamorra J, Thornton JG, Raine-Fenning N, Coomarasamy A. The prevalence of congenital uterine anomalies in unselected and high-risk populations: A systematic review. *Hum Reprod Update.* 2011;17:761–71.
5. The American Fertility Society classifications of adnexal adhesions, distal tubal obstruction, tubal occlusion secondary to tubal ligation, tubal pregnancies, Müllerian anomalies and intrauterine adhesions. *Fertil Steril.* 1988;49:944–55.
6. Randolph JF Jr, Ying YK, Maier DB, Schmidt CL, Riddick DH. Comparison of real-time ultrasonography, hysterosalpingography, and laparoscopy/hysteroscopy in the evaluation of uterine abnormalities and tubal patency. *Fertil Steril.* 1986;46:828–32.
7. Nicolini U, Bellotti M, Bonazzi B, Zamberletti D, Candiani GB. Can ultrasound be used to screen uterine malformations? *Fertil Steril.* 1987;47:89–93.
8. Fedele L, Ferrazzi E, Dorta M, Vercellini P, Candiani GB. Ultrasonography in the differential diagnosis of "double" uteri. *Fertil Steril.* 1988;50:361–4.
9. Pellerito JS, McCarthy SM, Doyle MB, Glickman MG, DeCherney AH. Diagnosis of uterine anomalies: Relative accuracy of MR imaging, endovaginal sonography, and hysterosalpingography. *Radiology* 1992;183:795–800.
10. Jurkovic D, Geipel A, Gruboeck K, Jauniaux E, Natucci M, Campbell S. Three-dimensional ultrasound for the assessment of uterine anatomy and detection of congenital anomalies: Comparison with hysterosalpingography and two-dimensional sonography. *Ultrasound Obstet Gynecol.* 1995;5:233–7.
11. Pascual MA, Alcázar JL, Graupera B, Pedrero C, Fernandez-Cid M, Hereter L. A simple method for excluding uterine canalization defects using two-dimensional ultrasound in infertile women. *J Reprod Med.* 2017;62:133–7.
12. Graupera B, Pascual MA, Hereter L et al. Accuracy of three-dimensional ultrasound compared with magnetic resonance imaging in diagnosis of Müllerian duct anomalies using ESHRE-ESGE consensus on the classification of congenital anomalies of the female genital tract. *Ultrasound Obstet Gynecol.* 2015;46:616–22.
13. Simon C, Martinez L, Pardo F, Tortajada M, Pellicer A. Müllerian defects in women with normal reproductive outcome. *Fertil Steril.* 1991;56:1192–3.
14. Puscheck EE, Cohen L. Congenital malformations of the uterus: The role of ultrasound. *Semin Reprod Med.* 2008;26:223–31.
15. Venetis CA, Papadopoulos SP, Campo R, Gordts S, Tarlatzis BC, Grimbizis GF. Clinical implications of congenital uterine anomalies: A meta-analysis of comparative studies. *Reprod Biomed Online.* 2014;29:665–83.
16. Hall-Craggs MA, Kirkham A, Creighton SM. Renal and urological abnormalities occurring with Müllerian anomalies. *J Pediatr Urol.* 2013;9:27–32.
17. Troiano RN, McCarthy SM. Müllerian duct anomalies: Imaging and clinical issues. *Radiology* 2004;233:19–34.
18. Bermejo C, Martínez Ten P, Cantarero R et al. Three-dimensional ultrasound in the diagnosis of Müllerian duct anomalies and concordance with magnetic resonance imaging. *Ultrasound Obstet Gynecol.* 2010;35:593–601.

19. Bermejo C, Martínez-Ten P, Recio M, Ruiz-López L, Díaz D, Illescas T. Three-dimensional ultrasound and magnetic resonance imaging assessment of cervix and vagina in women with uterine malformations. *Ultrasound Obstet Gynecol.* 2014;43:336–45.

20. Sampson JA. Peritoneal endometriosis due to the menstrual dissemination of endometrial tissue into the peritoneal cavity. *Am J Obstet Gynecol.* 1927;14:422–69.

21. Sanfilippo JS, Wakim NG, Schikler KN, Yussman MA. Endometriosis in association with uterine anomaly. *Am J Obstet Gynecol.* 1986;154:39–43.

22. Olive DL, Henderson DY. Endometriosis and Müllerian anomalies. *Obstet Gynecol.* 1987;69:412–5.

23. Nawroth F, Rahimi G, Nawroth C, Foth D, Ludwig M, Schmidt T. Is there an association between septate uterus and endometriosis? *Hum Reprod.* 2006;21:542–4.

24. LaMonica R, Pinto J, Luciano D, Lyapis A, Luciano A. Incidence of septate uterus in reproductive-aged women with and without endometriosis. *J Minim Invasive Gynecol.* 2016;23:610–3.

25. Leyendecker G, Kunz G, Wildt L, Beil D, Deininger H. Uterine hyperperistalsis and dysperistalsis as dysfunctions of the mechanism of rapid sperm transport in patients with endometriosis and infertility. *Hum Reprod.* 1996;11:1542–51.

26. Matalliotakis M, Goulielmos GN, Matalliotaki C, Trivli A, Matalliotakis I, Arici A. Endometriosis in adolescent and young girls: Report on a series of 55 cases. *J Pediatr Adolesc Gynecol.* 2017;30:568–70.

27. Zhang H, Qu H, Ning G, Cheng B, Jia F, Li X, Chen X. MRI in the evaluation of obstructive reproductive tract anomalies in paediatric patients. *Clin Radiol.* 2017;72:612.e7–612.e15.

28. Breech LL, Laufer MR. Müllerian anomalies. *Obstet Gynecol Clin N Am* 2009;36:47–68.

29. Junqueira BL, Allen LM, Spitzer RF, Lucco KL, Babyn PS, Doria AS. Müllerian duct anomalies and mimics in children and adolescents: Correlative intraoperative assessment with clinical imaging. *Radiographics* 2009;29:1085–103.

30. Cooper A, Merrit D. "Vulvovaginal and Müllerian anomalies." *Nelson Textbook of Pediatrics.* 19th ed. Kliegman R (ed). Philadelphia, PA. Elsevier. 2011, pp. 1874e1–e6.

31. Blask AR, Sanders RC, Rock JA. Obstructed uterovaginal anomalies: Demonstration with sonography. Part II. Teenagers. *Radiology.* 1991;179:84–88.

32. Vallerie AM, Breech LL. Update in Müllerian anomalies: Diagnosis, management, and outcomes. *Curr Opin Obstet Gynecol.* 2010;22:381–7.

33. Xie Z, Zhang X, Liu J, Zhang N, Xiao H, Liu Y, Li L, Liu X. Clinical characteristics of congenital cervical atresia based on anatomy and ultrasound: A retrospective study of 32 cases. *Eur J Med Res.* 2014;19:10.

34. Purslow CE. A case of unilateral hematocolpos, hematometra, and hematosalpinx [letter]. *J Obstet Gynecol Br Emp.* 1922;29:643.

35. Smith NA, Laufer MR. Obstructed hemivagina and ipsilateral renal anomaly (OHVIRA) syndrome: Management and follow-up. *Fertil Steril* 2007;87:918–22.

36. Shavell VI, Montgomery S, Johnson SC, Diamond MP, Berman JM. Complete septate uterus, obstructed hemivagina, and ipsilateral renal anomaly: Pregnancy course complicated by a rare urogenital anomaly. *Arch Gynecol Obstet* 2009;280:449–52.

37. Liu MM. Unicornuate uterus with rudimentary horn. *Int J Gynaecol Obstet.* 1994;44:149–53.

38. Heinonen PK. Unicornuate uterus and rudimentary horn. *Fertil Steril.* 1997;68:224–30.

39. Frontino G, Bianchi S, Ciappina N, Restelli E, Borruto F, Fedele L. The unicornuate uterus with an occult adenomyotic rudimentary horn. *J Minim Invasive Gynecol* 2009;16:622–5.

40. Reichman D, Laufer MR, Robinson BK. Pregnancy outcomes in unicornuate uteri: A review. *Fertil Steril.* 2009;90:1886–94.

41. Morcel K, Camborieux L, Programme de Recherches sur les Aplasies Müllériennes, Guerrier D. Mayer-Rokitansky-Küster-Hauser (MRKH) syndrome. *Orphanet J Rare Dis.* 2007;14(2):13.

42. Hall-Craggs MA, Williams CE, Pattison SH, Kirkham AP, Creighton SM. Mayer-Rokitansky-Küster-Hauser syndrome: Diagnosis with MR imaging. *Radiology* 2013;269:787–92.
43. Wang Y, Lu J, Zhu L, Sun Z, Jiang B, Feng F, Jin Z. Evaluation of Mayer-Rokitansky-Küster-Hauser syndrome with magnetic resonance imaging: Three patterns of uterine remnants and related anatomical features and clinical settings. *Eur Radiol.* 2017;27:5215–24.
44. Robert HG. [Septate uterus with blind cavity without hematometra]. *CR Soc Fr Gynecol.* 1969;39:767.
45. Maddukuri SB, Karegowda LH, Prakashini K, Kantipudi S. Robert's uterus: A rare congenital Müllerian duct anomaly causing haematometra. *BMJ Case Rep.* 2014;pii:bcr2014204489, doi: 10.1136/bcr-2014-204489.
46. Ludwin A, Ludwin I, Martins WP. Robert's uterus: Modern imaging techniques and ultrasound-guided hysteroscopic treatment without laparoscopy or laparotomy. *Ultrasound Obstet Gynecol.* 2016;48:526–9.
47. Di Spiezio Sardo A, Giampaolino P, Scognamiglio M, Varelli C, Nazzaro G, Mansueto G, Nappi C, Grimbizis GF. An exceptional case of complete septate uterus with unilateral cervical aplasia (class U2bC3V0/ESHRE/ESGE classification) and isolated Müllerian remnants: Combined hysteroscopic and laparoscopic treatment. *J Minim Invasive Gynecol.* 2016;23:16–17.
48. Lin PC. Reproductive outcomes in women with uterine anomalies. *J Womens Health (Larchmt).* 2004;13:33–39.
49. Nahum GG, Stanislaw H, McMahon C. Preventing ectopic pregnancies: How often does transperitoneal transmigration of sperm occur in effecting human pregnancy? *BJOG.* 2004;111:706–14.
50. Jayasinghe Y, Rane A, Stalewski H, Grover S. The presentation and early diagnosis of the rudimentary uterine horn. *Obstet Gynecol.* 2005;105:1456–67.
51. Nahum GG. Rudimentary uterine horn pregnancy: The 20th-century worldwide experience of 588 cases. *J Reprod Med.* 2002;47:151–63.
52. Tsafrir A, Rojansky N, Sela HY, Gomori JM, Nadjari M. Rudimentary horn pregnancy: First-trimester prerupture sonographic diagnosis and confirmation by magnetic resonance imaging. *J Ultrasound Med.* 2005;24:219–23.
53. Blancafort C, Graupera B, Pascual MÀ, Hereter L, Browne JL, Cusidó MT. Diagnosis and laparoscopic management of a rudimentary horn pregnancy: Role of three-dimensional ultrasound. *J Clin Ultrasound.* 2017;45:112–5.

CHAPTER 8

Pelvic Congestion Syndrome and Pelvic Adhesions

María Ángela Pascual and Jean L. Browne

INTRODUCTION

In this chapter, we will review the ultrasound findings of two causes of pelvic pain: pelvic congestion syndrome and pelvic adhesions.

PELVIC CONGESTION SYNDROME

Pelvic congestion is a known cause of chronic pelvic pain. It is usually associated with intrapelvic varicose veins in women with unexplained pain in the hypogastrium or pelvis that lasts more than 6 months. Pelvic congestion might also be seen with varicose vulvar veins, and associated with dyspareunia or postcoital pain.[1] However, numerous dilated intrapelvic varicose veins have also been reported in imaging studies of asymptomatic women.[2,3] In women with acute or subacute pelvic pain and negative findings in imaging studies, pain generally subsides or disappears. If present, pelvic congestion should not be regarded as the cause of acute or subacute pain.[4]

The nature of varicose pelvic veins is unknown, most certainly multifactorial, and due to mechanical and hormonal issues. Mechanical factors include the absence of valves in the ovarian veins. Compression of the retroaortic left renal vein between the aorta and the spine, or compression of the normal left renal vein by the aorto-superior mesenteric artery, is known as the nutcracker syndrome and causes retrograde venous stasis; these conditions may be diagnosed by abdominal ultrasound.[5-7] Compression of the left common iliac vein by the left main iliac artery, May-Thurner syndrome, is more frequent in women and may also cause pelvic veins congestion (Figure 8.1).[8] Estrogen influence leading to loose pelvic vein wall tension has been suggested to promote pelvic congestion syndrome.[9]

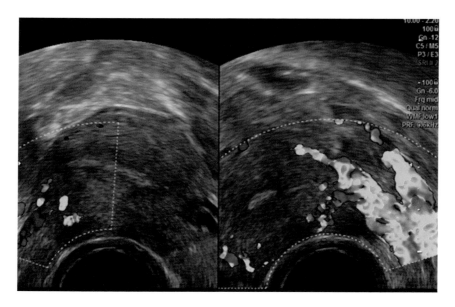

FIGURE 8.1   Images show left pelvic congestion. Note that the right vessels (image on the left) adjacent to the uterus show no congestion.

Endometriosis, large fibroids, or tumors may also engender secondary pelvic congestion (Figure 8.2).

The symptoms of pelvic congestion syndrome are borne by the mass effect that the varicose veins exert on the pelvic floor; they usually worsen during daily activity and while standing up, and may be relieved by lying down. The syndrome happens more often in middle-aged multiparous women due to the enlarged venous spaces and capacity of the pelvic venous system, the transitional weight increment, and the anatomic changes caused by pregnancy. The end result is vein dilatation (Figure 8.3) and tortuosity

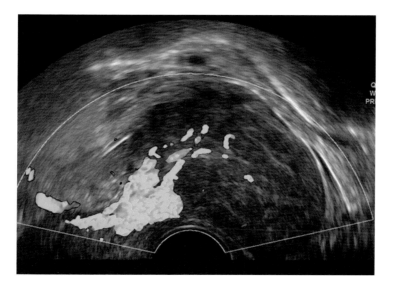

FIGURE 8.2   Large fibroids may also engender secondary pelvic congestion.

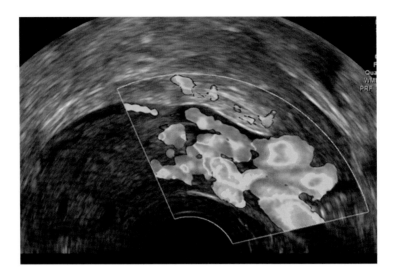

FIGURE 8.3   Color Doppler showing evident vein dilatation.

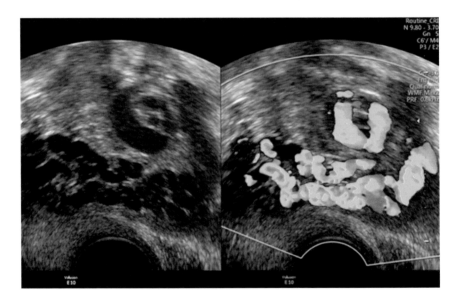

FIGURE 8.4   (Left) Sonogram shows dilated and tortuous vessels in gray scale. (Right) Doppler color confirms vascular congestion.

(Figures 8.4 and 8.5) that weigh on pelvic structures and lead to pelvic congestion syndrome symptomatology (Figure 8.6).[10] Thrombosis of the ovarian vein is a rare occurrence (Figures 8.7 through 8.11).[11]

Diagnosis may be achieved by many techniques. However, a good anamnesis and physical examination is paramount to choosing the most useful technique for each woman.[12,13] Imaging studies are used to identify the reasons that could lead to pelvic congestion syndrome or other diseases with which a differential diagnosis should be considered. Imaging with ultrasound with color Doppler (Figure 8.12), magnetic resonance imaging

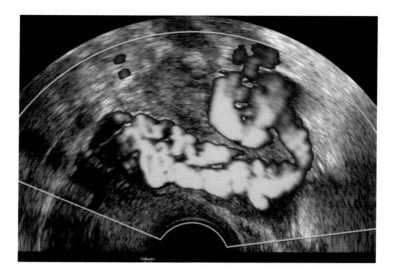

FIGURE 8.5   Same case as Figure 8.4 applying power Doppler.

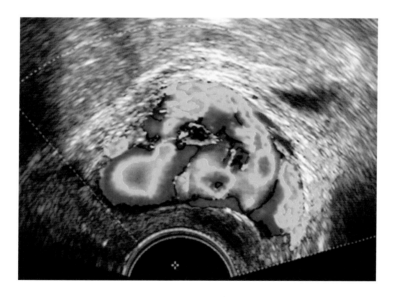

FIGURE 8.6   Evident pelvic congestion whose mass effect displaces pelvic organs.

(Figures 8.13 and 8.14), computed tomography (Figure 8.15), or phlebography may lead to the diagnosis. However, it must be kept in mind that since most of these tests are performed while lying down, venous changes and reflux may be decreased.[14]

Doppler ultrasound is widely used with good results (Figure 8.16).[15,16] Diagnostic criteria include ovarian vein diameter larger than 4 cm (Figure 8.17), dilated and tortuous arcuate uterine vessels (Figure 8.18), communication with varicose pelvic veins (Figure 8.19), slow venous flow, and retrograde venous reflux.

The diagnostic gold standard is MRI phlebography due to its high sensitivity.[17]

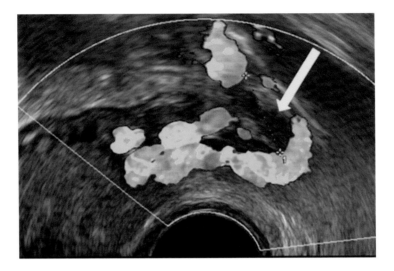

FIGURE 8.7   Color Doppler showing pelvic congestion. The yellow arrow indicates the presence of an intravascular thrombus.

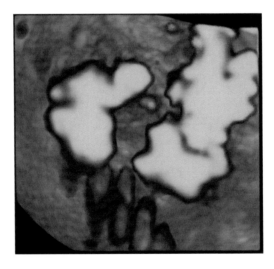

FIGURE 8.8   Same case as Figure 8.7, applying power Doppler clearly demonstrates the thrombus.

Short-term treatment of pelvic congestion syndrome starts with nonsteroidal anti-inflammatory medication to relieve pain. Medroxiprogestone[18] and Implanon[19] have been used with symptom relief in more than 50% of women in those studies.

Diagnostic criteria are technique dependent and treatment options for the pelvic congestion syndrome are limited. Some evidence points to a direct relationship between incompetent pelvic veins (IPV) and chronic pelvic pain (CPP) in women who have no other findings. Selective vein embolization with sclerosing substances should be a permanent solution. Venous embolization is safe and provides symptomatic relief in most women. However, results of many studies of embolization are hampered by a small number of cases, and the sole random study has been criticized for potential biases. The true relationship between IPV and CPP requires well-designed case control studies.[20]

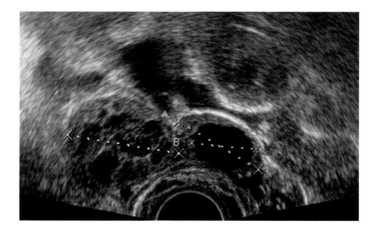

FIGURE 8.9   Right ovary with a growing follicle; to its left, a nodular septate cystic nodule is noticed. Histology revealed this to be an ovarian vein thrombosis.

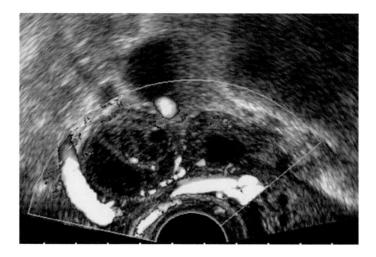

FIGURE 8.10   Same case as Figure 8.9. Power Doppler sonography demonstrated pelvic congestion and peripheral and central vascularization of the nodule (ovarian vein thrombosis).

PELVIC ADHESIONS

Adhesion syndrome or pelvic adhesions, also known as peritoneal inclusion cysts and benign cystic mesothelioma among other names (which are confusing but all related to the same disease),[21] is defined by symptoms and signs borne by intra-abdominal adhesions. Intraperitoneal adhesions are fibrous scar bands that develop between the surface of abdominal organs, tissues, and the peritoneum (Figure 8.20). Inflammation due to infection, surgery, endometriosis, or tumor disease may give rise to these scar bands.

Risk of adhesions is high after intestine surgery; appendicitis; or gynecologic surgery, such as hysterectomy (Figure 8.21),[22] myomectomy (Figure 8.22),[23] cesarean section,[24] or adnexal surgery. Radiotherapy on pelvic structures also risks engendering adhesions. Laparoscopic surgery is less prone to cause adhesions than laparotomy.

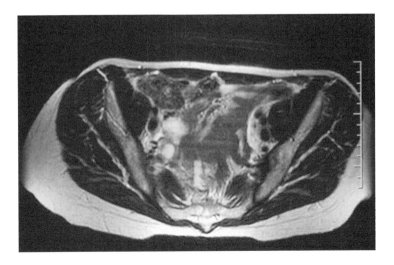

FIGURE 8.11   MRI contrast enhanced image shows hyperintense dilated right ovarian vein (same case as Figures 8.9 and 8.10).

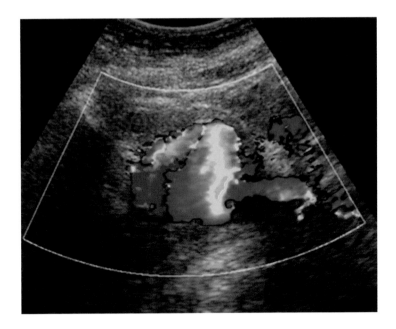

FIGURE 8.12   Vascular dilatation: incidental finding.

Loculation of peritoneal fluid by these fibrous bands determines the findings that describe adhesion syndrome (Figure 8.23).[25] Imaging of these findings may give rise to a wrong diagnosis, since their complexity may have them mistaken for benign or malignant ovarian cysts.[22,26]

Adhesions that compromise fallopian tubes may produce sterility or other reproduction anomalies[27,28] and may be diagnosed by ultrasound.

In 2004, Savelli et al.[21] described peritoneal pseudocyst ultrasound findings in 31 cases. The loculations of these pseudocysts usually have undefined margins and a complex

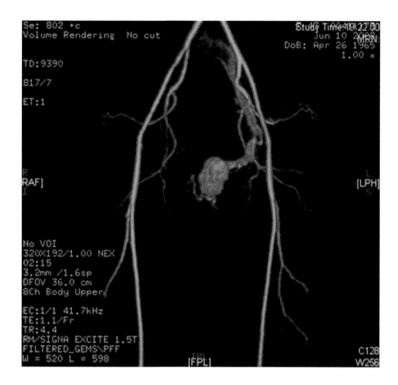

FIGURE 8.13   MR angiography: vascular shunt. Notice large left vein.

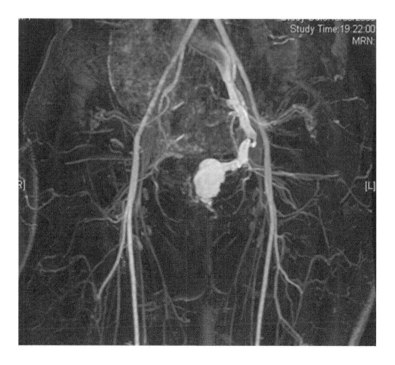

FIGURE 8.14   Same case as Figure 8.13. Arterial phase with early left vein visualization due to arteriovenous shunt.

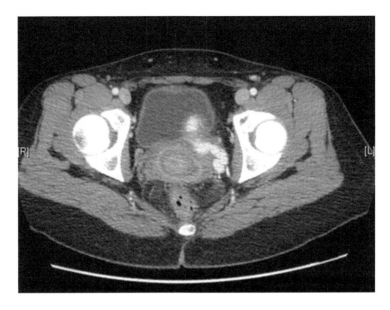

FIGURE 8.15   Same case as Figures 8.13 and 8.14. Note large left vein opacification in late arterial phase.

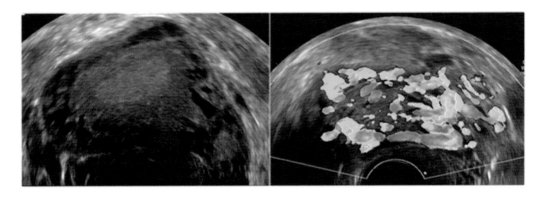

FIGURE 8.16   Ultrasound shows congestion of uterine and pelvic vessels in the postpartum period. (Left) Numerous dilated myometrial vessels. (Right) Color Doppler can provide a detailed demonstration of dilated vessels.

morphology (Figure 8.24), giving them a starlike (Figure 8.25), tubular (Figure 8.26), or clumping shape. Septa were present in 81% of cases and they are often shoved around while pushing the top of the vagina with the transvaginal probe during the ultrasound exploration. This has been described as the "flapping sail sign."[21]

Sayassneh and Ekechi et al. in 2015[29] described pseudocysts as multilocular cysts that are adherent to the ovarian surface (Figure 8.27). Septa are most frequently complete and thin, and generally move and "flap" when the cystic area is probed during transvaginal ultrasound (Figure 8.28). They have an irregular shape since they fill the pouch of Douglas and lie between the organs and structures of the pelvis, or may have a stellate or tubular form.[21,30] The cysts are generally anechoic, although they may also show low-level echogenicity content.[21]

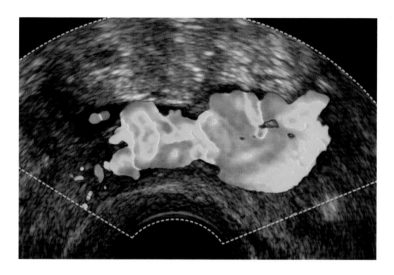

FIGURE 8.17   Sonogram showing the enlarged diameter of an ovarian vein.

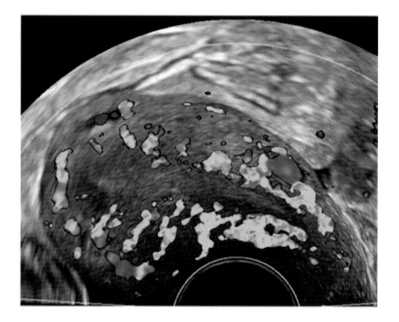

FIGURE 8.18   Sonogram demonstrating dilated and tortuous arcuate uterine vessels.

Pelvic adhesions may cause chronic or long-term pain. Adhesions that limit movement of pelvic structures and organs are painful, especially those that affect ovaries and fix the uterus and the omentum. Adhesions between the uterus and the ovary have been profusely described by various authors,[27,31–33] and are often related to the presence of endometriosis involvement of the ovary.

Nerves have been found in pelvic adhesions; however, they have not always been found in those of symptomatic patients. These findings suggest that adhesions go through different stages, leading to mature fibrous tissue with its own vessels and nerves.[34]

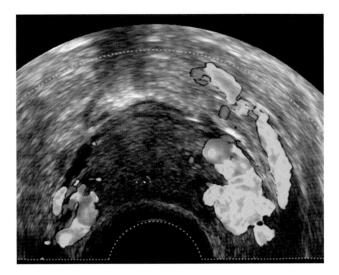

FIGURE 8.19   Dilated arcuate uterine vessels communicating with varicose pelvic veins.

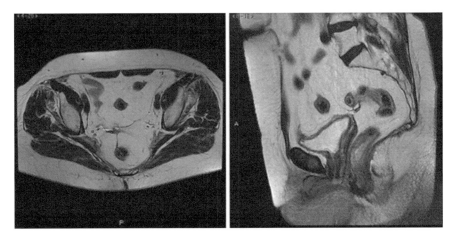

FIGURE 8.20   Thin postsurgical adhesions to bladder, sigmoid, and rectum following surgery for endometrial cancer. Images have been stable for more than 2 years.

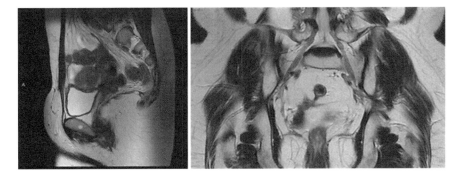

FIGURE 8.21   Thick postsurgical adhesions following hysterectomy of multiple intestinal loops at the vaginal stump.

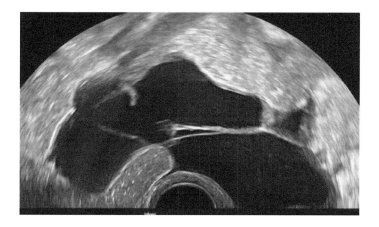

FIGURE 8.22   Sonogram showing thick adhesions after hysterectomy.

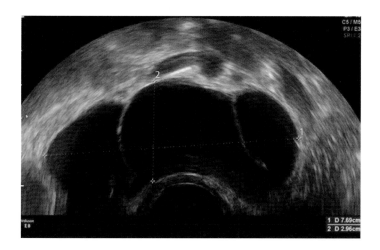

FIGURE 8.23   Image showing loculation of peritoneal fluid.

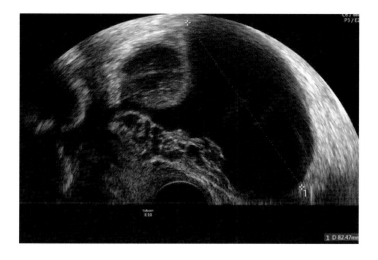

FIGURE 8.24   Sonogram showing a pseudocyst with a complex morphology.

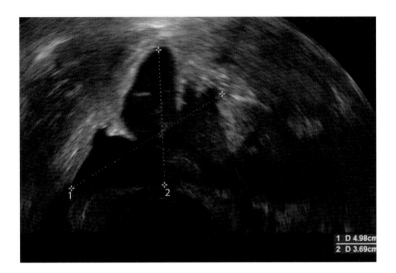

FIGURE 8.25   Pelvic adhesions with a starlike morphology.

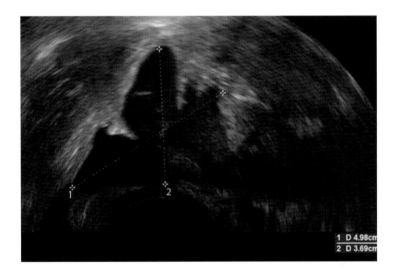

FIGURE 8.26   Example of adhesions of tubular morphology.

Controversy surrounds the relation between adhesions and chronic pelvic pain (CPP) since some studies found the same prevalence and distribution of pelvic adhesions in patients with CPP as in asymptomatic women with infertility. Also, laparoscopic adhesiolysis would be expected to allow pain to subside. There is only one randomized study of adhesiolysis versus no treatment, and after 16 months there were no clinical differences between both groups. Only patients who had thick, very vascular adhesions compromising the bladder had pain relief.[35]

There is also disagreement over treatment, since although laparoscopic adhesiolysis diminishes chronic abdominal pain, results of pain evolution are no better than with diagnostic laparoscopy alone.[36]

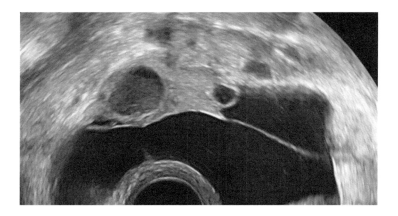

FIGURE 8.27   Sonogram showing multilocular pseudocyst adherent to the ovary surface.

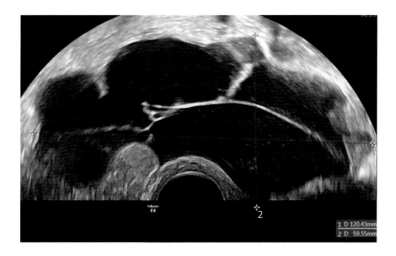

FIGURE 8.28   Pseudocyst showing complete thin septa, which have a wavelike motion when pushed by the probe: The "flapping sail sign."

ACKNOWLEDGMENTS

Written under the auspices of the Càtedra d' Investigació en Obstetrícia i Ginecologia de la Universitat Autònoma de Barcelona. Thanks to Beatriz Valero for help in the editing of this work.

REFERENCES

1. Zondervan KT, Yudkin PL, Vessey MP, Dawes MG, Barlow DH, Kennedy SH. Prevalence and incidence of chronic pelvic pain in primary care: Evidence from a national general practice database. *Br J Obstet Gynaecol.* 1999;106:1149–55.
2. Rozenblit AM, Ricci ZJ, Tuvia J, Amis ES Jr. Incompetent and dilated ovarian veins: A common CT finding in asymptomatic parous women. *AJR* 2001;176:119–22.
3. Hiromura T, Nishioka T, Nishioka S. Reflux in the left ovarian vein: Analysis of MDCT findings in asymptomatic women. *AJR* 2004;183:1411–5.
4. Harris RD, Holtzman SR, Poppe AM. Clinical outcome in female patients with pelvic pain and normal pelvic US findings. *Radiology* 2000;216:440–3.

5. Kim SH, Cho SW, Kim HD, Chung JW, Park JH, Han MC. Nutcracker syndrome: Diagnosis with Doppler US. *Radiology* 1996;198:93–97.

6. Bekou V, Zollikofer C, Nieuwkamp N, von Weymarn A, Duewell S, Traber J. A therapeutic option in nutcracker syndrome and ovarian vein insufficiency. *Phlebology* 2014;29:144–9.

7. Takebayashi S, Ueki T, Ikeda N, Fujikawa A. Diagnosis of the nutcracker syndrome with color Doppler sonography: Correlation with flow patterns on retrograde left renal venography. *AJR Am J Roentgenol.* 1999;172:39–43.

8. Kaltenmeier CT, Erben Y, Indes J, Lee A, Dardik A, Sarac T, Ochoa Chaar CI. Systematic review of May-Thurner syndrome with emphasis on gender differences. *J Vasc Surg Venous Lymphat Disord.* 2018;6:399–407.

9. Asciutto G, Mumme A, Asciutto KC, Geier B. Oestradiol levels in varicose vein blood of patients with and without pelvic vein incompetence (PVI): Diagnostic implications. *Eur J Vasc Endovasc Surg.* 2010;40:117–21.

10. Asciutto G, Mumme A, Asciutto KC, Geier B. Pelvic vein incompetence influences pain levels in patients with lower limb varicosity. *Phlebology* 2010;25:179–83.

11. Graupera B, Pascual MA, Garcia P, Di Paola R, Ubeda B, Tresserra F. Atypical ultrasonographic presentation of ovarian vein thrombosis. *Eur J Gynaec Oncol.* 2011;32:439–40.

12. van Os-Bossagh P, Pols T, Hop WC, Nelemans T, Erdmann W, Drogendijk AC, Bohnen AM. Questionnaire as diagnostic tool in chronic pelvic pain (CPP): A pilot study. *Eur J Obstet Gynecol Reprod Biol.* 2002;103:173–8.

13. O'Brien MT, Gillespie DL. Diagnosis and treatment of the pelvic congestion syndrome. *J Vasc Surg Venous Lymphat Disord.* 2015;3:96–106.

14. Asciutto G, Mumme A, Marpe B, Köster O, Asciutto KC, Geier B. MR venography in the detection of pelvic venous congestion. *Eur J Vasc Endovasc Surg.* 2008;36:491–6.

15. Creton D, Hennequin L, Kohler F, Allaert FA. Embolisation of symptomatic pelvic veins in women presenting with non-saphenous varicose veins of pelvic origin: Three-year follow-up. *Eur J Vasc Endovasc Surg.* 2007;34:112–7.

16. Liddle AD, Davies AH. Pelvic congestion syndrome: Chronic pelvic pain caused by ovarian and internal iliac varices. *Phlebology* 2007;22:100–4.

17. Meneses LQ, Uribe S, Tejos C, Andía ME, Fava M, Irarrazaval P. Using magnetic resonance phase-contrast velocity mapping for diagnosing pelvic congestion syndrome. *Phlebology* 2011;26:157–61.

18. Soysal ME, Soysal S, Vicdan K, Ozer S. A randomized controlled trial of goserelin and medroxyprogesterone acetate in the treatment of pelvic congestion. *Hum Reprod.* 2001;16:931–9.

19. Shokeir T, Amr M, Abdelshaheed M. The efficacy of Implanon for the treatment of chronic pelvic pain associated with pelvic congestion: 1-year randomized controlled pilot study. *Arch Gynecol Obstet.* 2009;280:437–43.

20. Champaneria R, Shah L, Moss J, Gupta JK, Birch J, Middleton LJ, Daniels JP. The relationship between pelvic vein incompetence and chronic pelvic pain in women: Systematic reviews of diagnosis and treatment effectiveness. *Health Technol Assess.* 2016;20:1–108.

21. Savelli L, De Iaco P, Ghi T, Bovicelli L, Rosati F, Cacciatore B. Transvaginal sonographic appearance of peritoneal pseudocysts. *Ultrasound Obstet Gynecol.* 2004;23:284–8.

22. Sohaey R, Gardner TL, Woodward PJ, Peterson M. Sonographic diagnosis of peritoneal inclusion cysts. *J Ultrasound Med.* 1995;14:913–7.

23. Ikechebelu JI, Eleje GU, Joe-Ikechebelu NN, Okafor CD, Akinobi AO. Comparison of the prevalence of adhesions at the time of diagnostic laparoscopy for infertility between patient who had open myomectomy and those who had no previous pelvic-abdominal surgery or pelvic inflammatory disease. *Niger J Clin Pract.* 2018;21:1415–21.

24. Dawood AS, Elgergawy AE. Incidence and sites of pelvic adhesions in women with post-caesarean infertility. *J Obstet Gynaecol.* 2018;8:1–6.

25. Koninckx PR, Renaer M, Brosens IA. Origin of peritoneal fluid in women: An ovarian exudation product. *Br J Obstet Gynaecol.* 1980;87:177–83.
26. Hoffer FA, Kozakewich H, Colodny A, Goldstein DP. Peritoneal inclusion cysts: Ovarian fluid in peritoneal adhesions. *Radiology* 1988;169:189–91.
27. Guerriero S, Ajossa S, Lai MP, Mais V, Paoletti AM, Melis GB. Transvaginal ultrasonography in the diagnosis of pelvic adhesions. *Hum Reprod.* 1997;12:2649–53.
28. Shalev J, Mashiach R, Fisch B, Royburt M, Bar-Hava I, Krissi H, Meizner I. Sonographic diagnosis of pelvic adhesions in patients after ovum pickup. *J Ultrasound Med.* 2001;20:869–75.
29. Sayasneh A, Ekechi CH, Ferrara L, Kaijser J, Stalder C, Sur S, Timmerman D, Bourne T. The characteristic ultrasound features of specific types of ovarian pathology (Review). *Int J Oncol.* 2015;46:445–58.
30. Jain AK. Imaging of peritoneal inclusion cysts. *AJR Am J Roentgenol.* 2000;174:1559–63.
31. Valentin L. Imaging in gynecology. *Best Prac Res Clin Obstet Gynaecol.* 2006;20:881–906.
32. Okaro E, Condous G, Khalid A, Timmerman D, Ameye L, Huffel SV, Bourne T. The use of ultrasound based "soft markers" for the prediction of pelvic pathologyin women with chronic pelvic pain—Can we reduce the need for laparoscopy? *Br J Obstet Gynaecol.* 2006;113:251–6.
33. Guerriero S, Ajossa S, Garau N, Alcázar JL, Mais V, Melis GB. Diagnosis of pelvic adhesions in patients with endometrioma; the role of tranvaginal ultrasonography. *Fertil Steril.* 2010;94:742–6.
34. Kligman I, Drachenberg C, Papadimitriou J, Katz E. Immunohistochemical demonstration of nerve fibers in pelvic adhesions. *Obstet Gynecol.* 1993;82:566–8.
35. Howard FM, El-Minawi AM, Sanchez RA. Conscious pain mapping by laparoscopy in women with chonic pelvic pain. *Obstet Gynecol.* 2000;96:934–9.
36. Swank DJ, Swank-Bordewijk SC, Hop WC, van Erp WF, Janssen IM, Bonjer HJ, Jeekel J. Laparoscopic adhesiolysis in patients with chronic abdominal pain: A blinded randomised controlled multi-centre trial. *Lancet* 2003;361:1247–51.

CHAPTER 9

Non-Gynecological Causes of Pelvic Pain

Juan Luis Alcázar

INTRODUCTION

Pelvic pain is a common complaint in women of all ages and may be due to many different causes. Whatever the cause of the pain, a thorough clinical history and physical examination is mandatory. Pelvic pain may be acute or chronic.[1]

Ultrasound, either transabdominal, transvaginal, or transrectal, is considered the imaging modality of choice for evaluating women with pelvic pain because of lack of ionizing radiation, low cost, and widespread availability.[2]

Previous chapters of this book addressed the ultrasound findings for most gynecological causes of pelvic pain in women. However, gynecologists should also bear in mind that there are other causes from non-gynecologic origin. This is essential for a correct differential diagnosis. An apparent "normal gynecologic scan" should not preclude searching for other potential causes of pelvic pain not related to the internal genital organs, such as appendicitis, ureteric calculi, bladder lesions, diverticulitis, urethral lesions, vascular lesions, and non-gynecologic pelvis neoplasms.

In this chapter, we will review the clinical use of pelvic ultrasound scan (transabdominal, transvaginal, or transrectal routes) for evaluating non-gynecological causes of pelvic pain in women.

ACUTE APPENDICITIS

The evaluation of non-pregnant women presenting with acute right lower quadrant abdominal pain remains a clinical challenge. Acute appendicitis, right ureteric calculi, and adnexal pathology are the main entities causing this type of pain. Clinical manifestations may be similar in all these entities, including acute onset pain with variable intensity, often associated with nausea, vomiting, leukocytosis, and fever.[1]

The estimated lifetime risk for appendicitis in women is 6.7%, being more frequent in women age 15–19 years old, but appendicitis may occur in women at any age.[3]

Due to the relatively nonspecific clinical presentation, imaging techniques have become essential in the diagnosis of appendicitis. Transabdominal ultrasound has been reported as having a 80%–94% sensitivity for detecting acute appendicitis when the appendix is seen as a blind-ended, noncompressible, aperistaltic tubular structure arising from the base of the cecum and with a diameter >6 mm (Figure 9.1).[4] A recent meta-analysis has shown that pooled sensitivity of ultrasound is 86% and pooled specificity is 91%.[5] False negative cases usually occur in the retrocecal position of the appendix.[4]

Discontinuity in the echogenic submucosa is suggestive of impending perforation. If perforation occurs, a localized periappendiceal abscess may be seen (Figure 9.2).[4] In some cases, appendicolith may be seen inside the appendix (Figure 9.3).

There are some reports about the use of transvaginal ultrasound for assessing acute appendicitis. Albeit there are no reports about the use of transrectal ultrasound in appendicitis, this approach could be considered for girls and adolescents. The ultrasound findings for acute appendicitis as observed by transvaginal ultrasound are quite similar to those observed by transabdominal ultrasound (Figure 9.4).[6–10] In addition, some authors have also reported that by using this technique, hyperemia of the appendix may also be a finding.

Molander et al. reported ultrasound findings from a case series of 31 women with clinical suspicion of pelvic inflammatory disease.[6] Six of them were ultimately diagnosed as having acute appendicitis by way of laparoscopic evaluation. They observed that ultrasound findings in these six women were suggestive of acute appendicitis and clearly different from those who had acute pelvic inflammatory disease.

Caspi et al. reported a series of 38 women with final histological diagnosis of acute appendicitis.[7] All these women underwent transabdominal and transvaginal ultrasound prior to surgery. These authors found that transabdominal ultrasound detected the inflamed appendix in 29 women (76%), but it was detected only by transvaginal ultrasound in 9 women (24%), highlighting the relevance of performing transvaginal ultrasound in women with suspected acute appendicitis and negative findings on transabdominal ultrasound. This may happen in the "pelvic appendix."[4]

Computed tomography scan (CT scan) and magnetic resonance imaging (MRI) are considered as second-line imaging techniques for assessing female patients presenting with suspected appendicitis.[1] CT scan and MRI findings for acute appendicitis are similar to those described for ultrasound: inflamed appendix, inflamed peri-appendiceal fat, appendicoliths, and appendix diameter >6 mm.[1,11] A recent meta-analysis has shown that diagnostic performance of CT scan and MRI after inconclusive ultrasound evaluation are similar in children and adult patients (Table 9.1).[12]

DIVERTICULITIS

Acute diverticulitis usually presents as a left lower quadrant pain and tenderness with elevated count and fever.[13] Acute diverticulitis occurs in up to 1.9% of women with diverticular disease. Most patients are in their fifth or sixth decade of life with an average

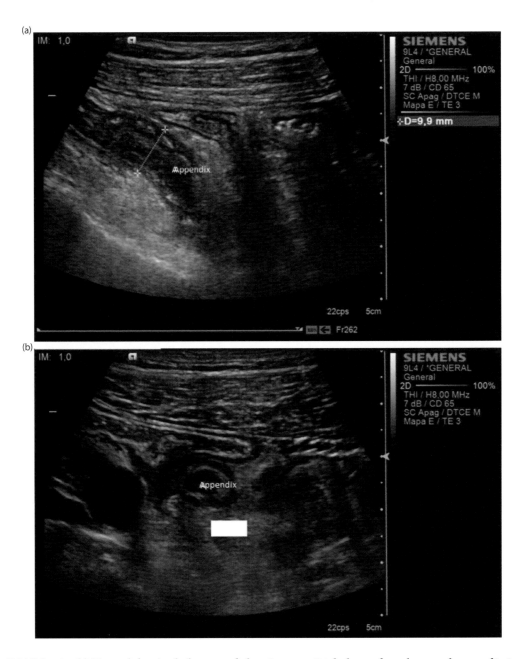

FIGURE 9.1   (a) Transabdominal ultrasound showing a sagittal plane of an abnormal appendix in a case of acute appendicitis. Note diameter: 9.9 mm. (b) Transverse plane.

age of 57.6 years old.[14] Most cases involve the rectosigmoid colon, but it may also affect any part of the bowel.[13]

Imaging diagnosis of acute diverticulitis is usually based on CT scan findings. The most sensitive signs for acute diverticulitis on CT scan are bowel wall thickening and fat stranding (Figure 9.5).[15] Wall thickness is >4 mm in large bowel and >3 mm in small bowel. Accuracy for CT scan has been reported to be as high as 98%.[16,17]

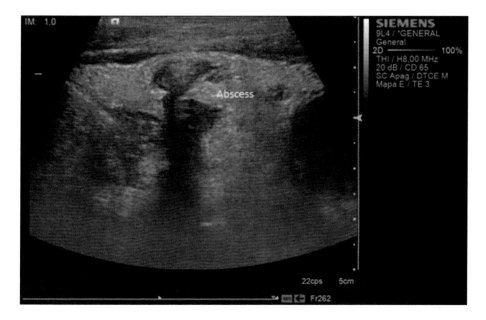

FIGURE 9.2   Transabdominal ultrasound showing a case of appendicitis with periappendicular abscess.

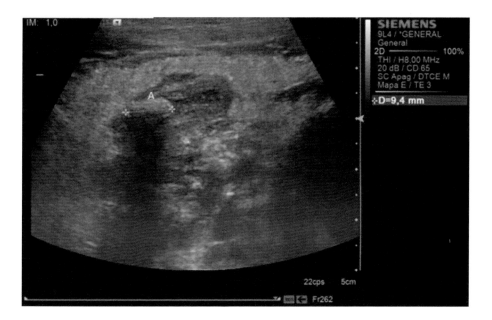

FIGURE 9.3   Transabdominal ultrasound showing a case of appendicitis. An appendicolith is observed (A).

Ultrasound also has a role for diagnosing acute diverticulitis. Ultrasound findings suggestive of acute diverticulitis include bowel wall thickening, pericolic inflammation, and inflamed diverticulum (Figure 9.6).[15] Transvaginal ultrasound may be useful in some cases, especially when diverticula are lying down in the pelvis.[4]

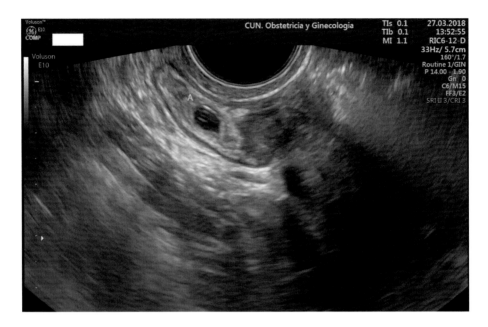

FIGURE 9.4   A case of acute appendicitis as observed by transvaginal ultrasound. The appendix is observed thickened (A).

TABLE 9.1   Diagnostic Performance of CT Scan and MRI for Diagnosing Appendicitis

	Sensitivity (%)	Specificity (%)
CT Scan		
Children	96.2	94.6
Adults	89.9	93.6
MRI		
Children	97.4	97.1
Adults	89.9	93.6

A meta-analysis reported in 2008 showed that both CT scan and ultrasound had similar diagnostic performance in terms of sensitivity (92% for ultrasound versus 94% for CT scan) and specificity (90% for ultrasound versus 99% for CT scan).[18]

BOWEL INFLAMMATORY DISEASE

Crohn's disease is a chronic, granulomatous inflammatory process that affects the bowel. This disease may be a cause of pelvic pain that affects the rectosigmoid colon and mostly young patients. Ultrasound may help to diagnose Crohn's disease.[4] Bowel wall thickening, inflammation of the mesenteric fat, strictures, and even fistulas may be detected by ultrasound. Pelvic abscesses may also be observed.[4]

URETERIC CALCULI

Ultrasound has shown high sensitivity for detecting renal calculi.[4] However, most ureteric calculi are located in the distal ureter in the ureterovesical junction.[19] Transabdominal

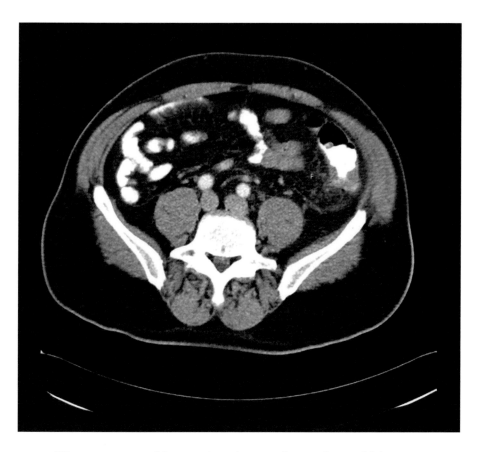

FIGURE 9.5 CT scan in a case of diverticulitis. Fat stranding is observed (F).

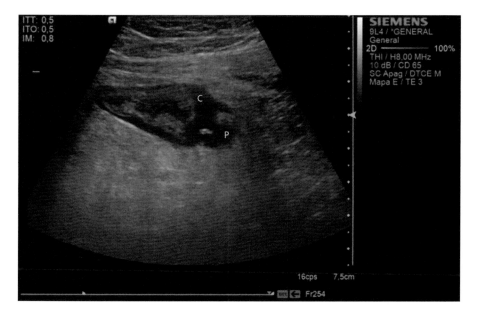

FIGURE 9.6 Transabdominal ultrasound in a case of acute diverticulitis. One can observe wall thickening of the colon (C) and pericolonic inflammation (P).

ultrasound allows detection of many calculi at the intramural ureter. However, in some cases overdistention of the bladder may cause distal displacement of the trigone, making it difficult to visualize the stone.[4]

The intramural ureter can be easily visualized by transvaginal ultrasound, with a visualization rate reported as high as 93%.[20]

The technique we use is as follows: The bladder should not be totally empty. First, the ureteral meatus should be located at the level of the bladder wall, slightly protruding into the bladder lumen by displacing the transvaginal transducer backward and laterally (Figure 9.7), then the transducer is displaced laterally and anteriorly at the same time that it is rotated internally, then the ureter can be visualized as a hypoechoic band within the bladder wall (Figure 9.8). The visualization of the ureteral jet may help to identify the ureteral meatus (Figure 9.9).

The ureteric calculi are usually seen as hyperechoic round or oval lesions with acoustic shadowing (Figures 9.10 through 9.12).

Early reports showed that transvaginal ultrasound might be an excellent tool for detecting ureteric stones in the distal ureter, particularly if the results of transabdominal ultrasound are normal or inconclusive. Laing et al. showed that transvaginal ultrasound detected ureteric calculi in all cases in a case series of 13 women with clinical suspicion of ureterolithiasis. Transabdominal ultrasound was only detected in 2 out of 13 cases.[21]

Yang et al. reported a retrospective study involving 7 women with distal ureteric stones and 20 controls.[22] They evaluated the height of the ureteral papilla (meatus) in both groups. They reported an interesting finding: The height of the ureteral papilla from the involved ureter was significantly higher than the contralateral ureteral papilla and from ureteral papilla from controls (median height 6.7 versus 3.5 mm).

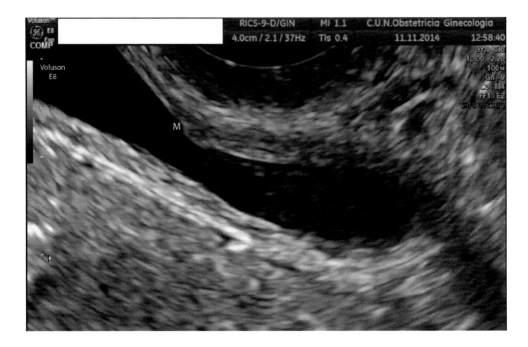

FIGURE 9.7   Transvaginal ultrasound showing the ureteral meatus (M).

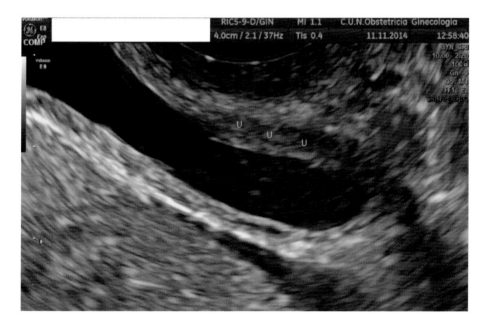

FIGURE 9.8   Transvaginal ultrasound showing the ureter (U) within the bladder wall.

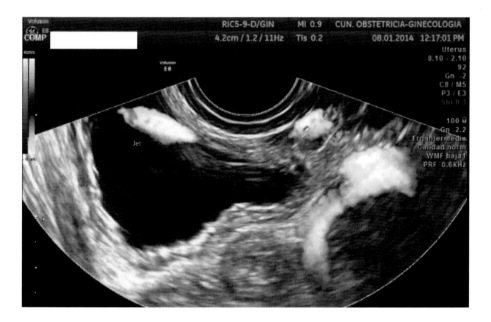

FIGURE 9.9   Transvaginal ultrasound showing the urine jet.

Mitterberger et al. reported on a prospective study of 62 women with clinical suspicion of ureterolithiasis, comparing the detection rate of intravenous urography, transabdominal ultrasound, and three-dimensional transrectal/transvaginal ultrasound.[23] Distal ureterolithiasis was confirmed in 55 women (ureterorenoscopy). The detection rate for intravenous urography, transabdominal ultrasound, and three-dimensional transrectal/ transabdominal ultrasound was 71%, 55%, and 100%, respectively.

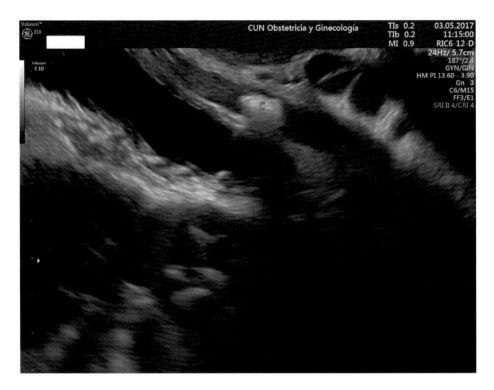

FIGURE 9.10   Transvaginal ultrasound showing a calculus (C) within the ureter.

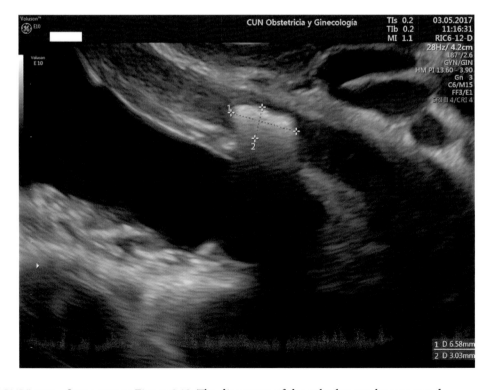

FIGURE 9.11   Same case as Figure 9.10. The diameters of the calculus can be measured.

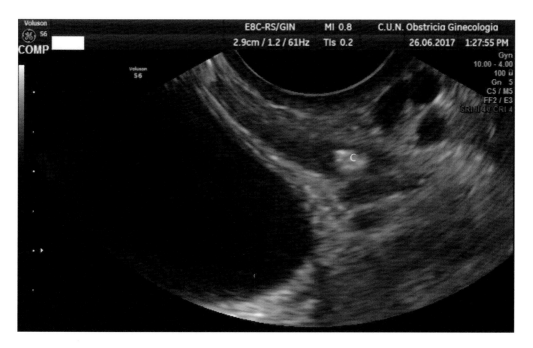

FIGURE 9.12   Another ureteric calculus (C) as detected by transvaginal ultrasound.

More recently, Holland et al. reported a retrospective series of 5594 women presenting with pelvic pain at their institution.[24] All women underwent transvaginal ultrasound according to a predefined scanning protocol that included systematic assessment of the distal ureter. Seven women (0.1%) had ureteric stones. All of them were detected by transvaginal ultrasound.

They concluded that distal ureter assessment by transvaginal ultrasound should be part of the standard evaluation in women presenting with pelvic pain at a gynecologic clinic.

BLADDER LESIONS

Bladder lesions are not a frequent cause of pelvic pain. However, for any woman presenting with hypogastric pain, assessment of the bladder is advisable. Transvaginal ultrasound is an optimal tool for assessing the bladder. A moderate to small amount of urine is required for assessing the bladder and the urethra. The transducer should be orientated anteriorly and partial withdrawal is recommended.[4]

Different types of lesions can be detected, such as polyps (Figure 9.13), cancer (Figure 9.14), ureteroceles (Figure 9.15), endometriotic nodules (Figure 9.16), and urethral lesions (Figures 9.17 and 9.18).

In some cases, urethral slings may perforate the bladder, being a cause of pelvic pain (Figure 9.19).

PELVIC CONGESTION SYNDROME

Pelvic congestion syndrome is a clinical entity that may cause chronic pelvic pain. It is characterized by the presence of varicose veins in the pelvis, mostly involving the uterine

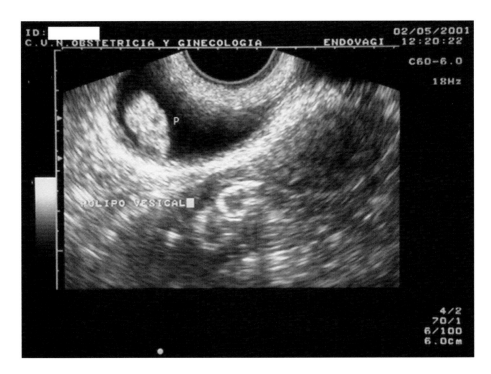

FIGURE 9.13   Transvaginal ultrasound showing a bladder polyp (P).

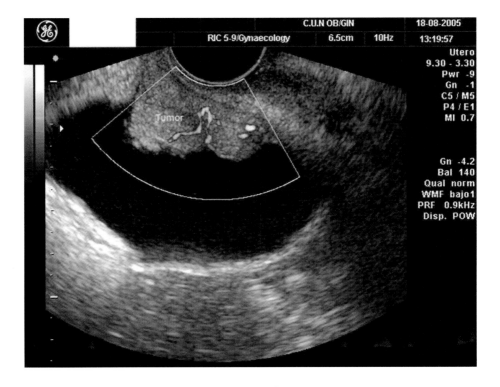

FIGURE 9.14   Transvaginal ultrasound showing bladder cancer.

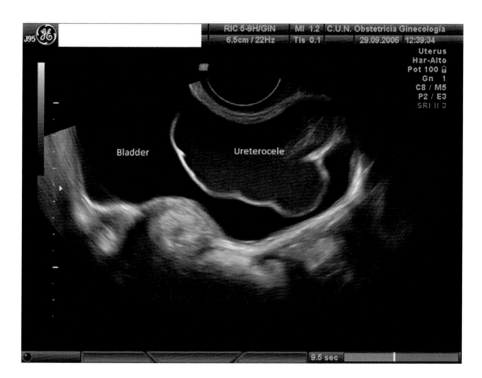

FIGURE 9.15   Transvaginal ultrasound showing an ureterocele.

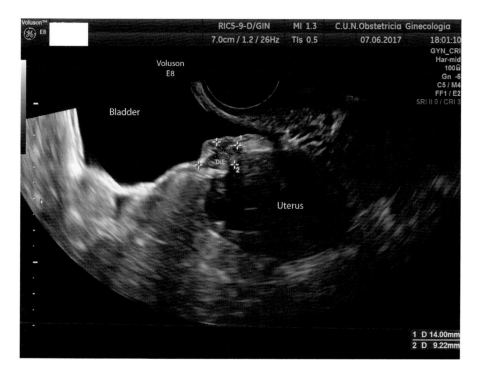

FIGURE 9.16   Transvaginal ultrasound showing an endometriotic nodule (DIE) involving the bladder wall.

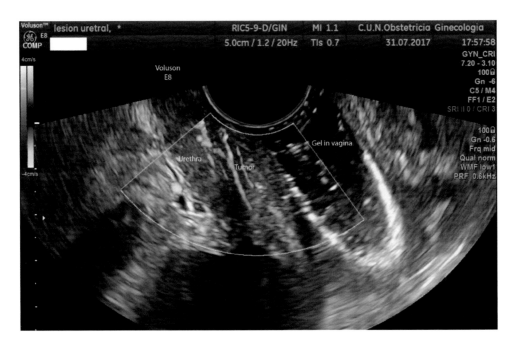

FIGURE 9.17   Transvaginal ultrasound showing a urethral tumor.

venous plexus. The main cause of pelvic congestion syndrome is incompetence of ovarian and uterine veins.

Phlebography is considered the reference standard technique for diagnosing pelvic venous disorders.[25] However, this technique is invasive and exposes the pelvis to ionizing radiation. For this reason, other imaging techniques, such as ultrasound, have emerged.

Ultrasound features of pelvic congestion syndrome are mainly the presence of dilated veins around the uterus (the so-called pelvic varicocele).[26] These dilated veins are usually observed as multiple anechoic areas that may resemble a multilocular adnexal cyst. The use of color or power Doppler is very helpful since these lacunae fill with Doppler signals (Figure 9.20). Another finding is the dilatation of the left ovarian vein (usually a diameter >6–7 mm).[26]

MRI and CT scan have also been proposed for evaluating women with pelvic congestion syndrome.[27]

A recent meta-analysis has shown that ultrasound has a similar diagnostic performance to MRI in terms of sensitivity (91%–100% for ultrasound and 88% for MRI) and specificity (100% for ultrasound and 100% for MRI).[28]

Due to the lower cost and wider availability, ultrasound should be the preferred technique.

PELVIC TUMORS OF NON-GYNECOLOGIC ORIGIN

In the pelvis, there is a wide range of different benign and malignant tumors not originating in the uterus and adnexa. Many of them may present with pelvic pain. Gynecologists evaluating female patients with pelvic pain should be aware of these tumors. We will review the sonographic features of some pelvic tumors from a non-gynecologic origin.

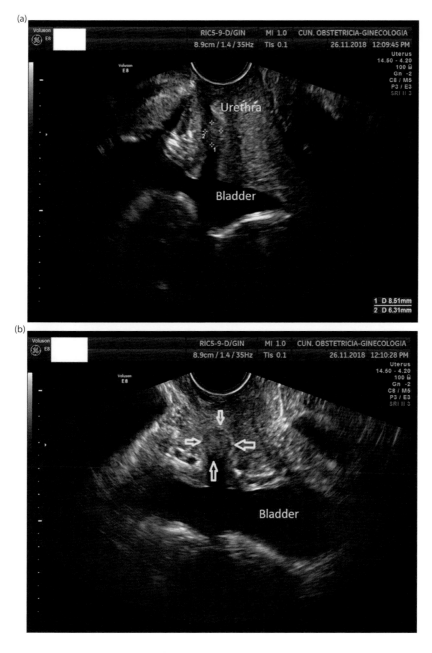

FIGURE 9.18 Transvaginal ultrasound showing a urethral polyp in the (a) sagittal plane and (b) transverse plane.

Rectal-Sigmoid Cancer

There are reports of cases of rectal tumors detected by transvaginal or transrectal ultrasound.[29] The typical ultrasound features are solid masses with irregular contours that are moderately or highly vascularized detected within the lumen of the rectum or sigmoid colon (Figure 9.21).

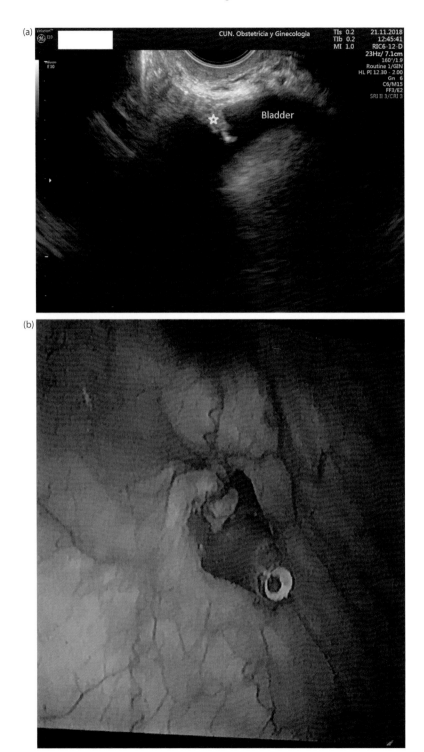

FIGURE 9.19   (a) Transvaginal ultrasound showing a urethral sling perforating the bladder. (b) Confirmed at cystoscopy.

(a)
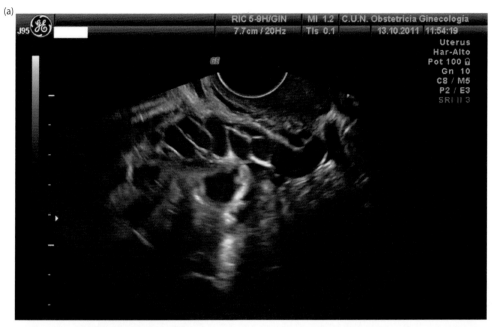

(b)
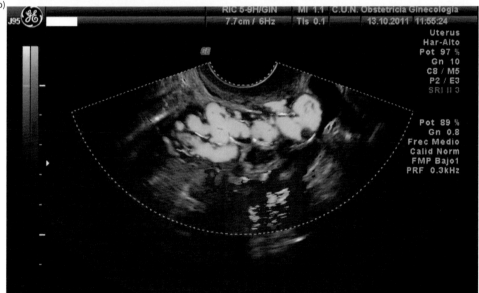

FIGURE 9.20 (a) Transvaginal ultrasound showing an elongated multilocular cystic structure. (b) Power Doppler depicts this structure corresponding to the venous pelvic varicocele.

Mucocele of the Appendix

Appendiceal mucocele is a cystic dilatation of the appendix due to accumulation of gelatinous mucoid material within the lumen. The reported incidence is low (0.2%–0.3%).[30] The ultrasound features of mucocele of the appendix include an elongated unilocular cystic structure with mixed echogenic content (Figure 9.22).[30] Differential diagnosis with other gynecologic tumors should be done.

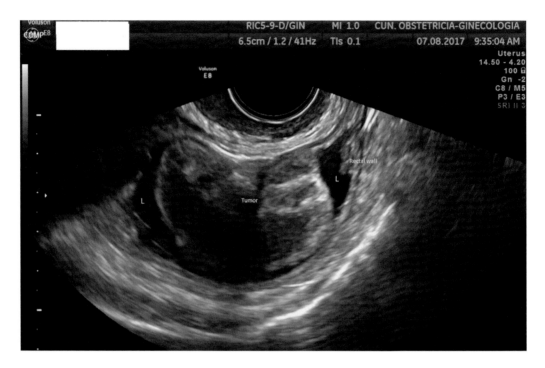

FIGURE 9.21   Transvaginal ultrasound showing a rectal cancer. L, rectal lumen.

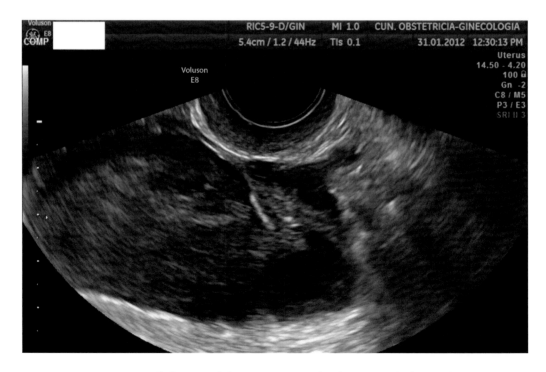

FIGURE 9.22   Transvaginal ultrasound showing an appendicular mucocele depicted as an elongated unilocular cystic structure with mixed echogenic content.

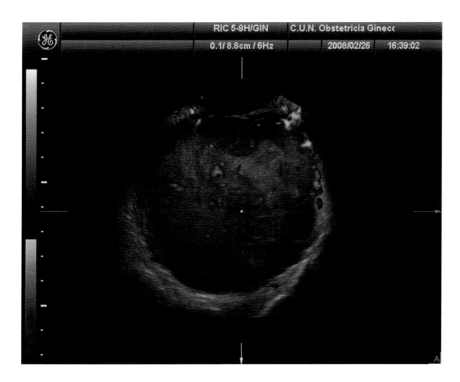

FIGURE 9.23   Transvaginal ultrasound showing a gastrointestinal stromal tumor depicted as a solid heterogeneous mass with moderate vascularization.

Gastrointestinal Stromal Tumors

Gastrointestinal stromal tumors (GISTs) are uncommon, accounting for 0.1%–1% of all gastrointestinal malignancies.[31] Most patients are older than 40 years old, being uncommon in young women. Ultrasound features of GIST include the presence of a solid heterogeneous mass with moderate or abundant vascularization (Figure 9.23).[32,33] Differential diagnosis with other gynecologic tumors should be done.

Pelvic Schwannoma

Schwannomas are tumors of neurogenic origin arising from nerve sheaths. Pelvic schwannomas account for 1%–3% of all schwannomas.[34] They most frequently affect females in their second to fifth decades of life.[35] There are some reports of ultrasound features of pelvic schwannomas. These tumors usually appear as large multilocular cystic masses (Figure 9.24).[34-36] Differential diagnosis with other pelvis gynecologic tumors should be done.

Pelvic Lymphocele

Pelvic lymphocele is a complication that occurs after lymphadenectomy for gynecological or urological malignancy, or after renal transplantation. The estimated prevalence of lymphocele after lymphadenectomy in gynecological oncologic surgery is about 20%, with 6% of them being symptomatic (pelvic pain).[37]

The typical ultrasound appearance of pelvic lymphocele is the presence of a well-defined round or oval thin-walled and smooth cyst located over the iliac vessels (Figure 9.25).[37]

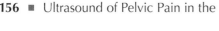

FIGURE 9.24 Transvaginal ultrasound showing a schwannoma depicted as a large multilocular cystic mass.

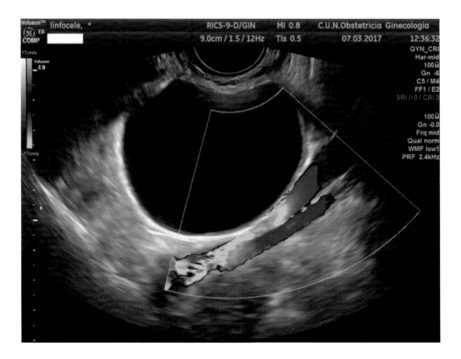

FIGURE 9.25 Transvaginal ultrasound showing a pelvic lymphocele depicted as a cystic anechoic lesion over the external iliac vessels.

This type of lesion should be considered in women presenting with pelvic pain after gynecological oncologic surgery. Transvaginal ultrasound is excellent for its diagnosis.

Differential diagnosis with other simple cysts within the pelvis should be made, especially if adnexa have not been removed during surgery.

REFERENCES

1. Amirbekian S, Hooley RJ. Ultrasound evaluation of pelvic pain. *Radiol Clin North Am.* 2014;52:1215–35.
2. Bhosale PR, Javitt MC Atri M et al. ACR Appropriateness Criteria® acute pelvic pain in the reproductive age group. *Ultrasound Q.* 2016;32:108–15.
3. Addiss DG, Shaffer N, Fowler BS, Tauxe RV. The epidemiology of apendicitis and appendectomy in the United States. *Am J Epidemiol.* 1990;132:910–25.
4. Damani N, Wilson SR. Nongynecologic applications of transvaginal US. *Radiographics.* 1999;19:S179–200.
5. Benabbas R, Hanna M, Shah J, Sinert R. Diagnostic accuracy of history, physical examination, laboratory tests, and point-of-care ultrasound for pediatric acute appendicitis in the emergency department: A systematic review and meta-analysis. *Acad Emerg Med.* 2017;24:523–51.
6. Molander P, Paavonen J, Sjöberg J, Savelli L, Cacciatore B. Transvaginal sonography in the diagnosis of acute appendicitis. *Ultrasound Obstet Gynecol.* 2002;20:496–501.
7. Caspi B, Zbar AP, Mavor E, Hagay Z, Appelman Z. The contribution of transvaginal ultrasound in the diagnosis of acute appendicitis: An observational study. *Ultrasound Obstet Gynecol.* 2003;21:273–6.
8. Bramante R, Radomski M, Nelson M, Raio C. Appendicitis diagnosed by emergency physician performed point-of-care transvaginal ultrasound: Case series. *West J Emerg Med.* 2013;14:415–8.
9. Haider Z, Condous G, Ahmed S, Kirk E, Bourne T. Transvaginal sonographic diagnosis of appendicitis in acute pelvic pain. *J Ultrasound Med.* 2006;25:1243–4.
10. Al-Roubaie M, Pellerito J. Findings of acute appendicitis on transvaginal ultrasound. *Ultrasound Q.* 2014;30:213–5.
11. Knoepp US, Mazza MB, Chong ST, Wasnik AP. MR Imaging of pelvic emergencies in women. *Magn Reson Imaging Clin N Am.* 2017;25:503–19.
12. Eng KA, Abadeh A, Ligocki C, Lee YK, Moineddin R, Adams-Webber T, Schuh S, Doria AS. Acute Appendicitis: A meta-analysis of the diagnostic accuracy of US, CT, and MRI as second-line imaging tests after an initial US. *Radiology* 2018;288:717–27.
13. Ellison DL. Acute diverticulitis management. *Crit Care Nurs Clin North Am.* 2018;30:67–74.
14. McConnell EJ, Tessier DJ, Wolff BG. Population-based incidence of complicated diverticular disease of the sigmoid colon based on gender and age. *Dis Colon Rectum.* 2003;46:1110–4.
15. Kandagatla PG, Stefanou AJ. Current status of the radiologic assessment of diverticular disease. *Clin Colon Rectal Surg.* 2018;31:217–20.
16. Werner A, Diehl SJ, Farag-Soliman M, Düber C. Multi-slice spiral CT in routine diagnosis of suspected acute left-sided colonic diverticulitis: A prospective study of 120 patients. *Eur Radiol.* 2003;13:2596–603.
17. Ambrosetti P, Becker C, Terrier F. Colonic diverticulitis: Impact of imaging on surgical management—A prospective study of 542 patients. *Eur Radiol.* 2002;12:1145–9.
18. Laméris W, van Randen A, Bipat S, Bossuyt PM, Boermeester MA, Stoker J. Graded compression ultrasonography and computed tomography in acute colonic diverticulitis: Meta-analysis of test accuracy. *Eur Radiol.* 2008;18:2498–511.
19. Yaqoob J, Usman MU, Bari V, Munir K, Mosharaf F. Unenhanced helical CT of ureterolithiasis: Incidence of secondary urinary tract findings. *J Pak Med Assoc.* 2004;54:2–5.

20. Pateman K, Mavrelos D, Hoo WL, Holland T, Naftalin J, Jurkovic D. Visualization of ureters on standard gynecological transvaginal scan: A feasibility study. *Ultrasound Obstet Gynecol.* 2013;41:696–701.

21. Laing FC, Benson CB, DiSalvo DN, Brown DL, Frates MC, Loughlin KR. Distal ureteral calculi: Detection with vaginal US. *Radiology* 1994;192:545–8.

22. Yang JM, Yang SH, Huang WC. Transvaginal sonography in the assessment of distal ureteral calculi. *Ultrasound Obstet Gynecol.* 2005;26:658–62.

23. Mitterberger M, Pinggera GM, Maier E, Neuwirt H, Neururer R, Pallwein L, Gradl J, Bartsch G, Strasser H, Frauscher F. Value of 3-dimensional transrectal/transvaginal sonography in diagnosis of distal ureteral calculi. *J Ultrasound Med.* 2007;26:19–27.

24. Holland T, Pateman K, Knez J, Dardelis G, Foo X, Jurkovic D. Diagnosis of distal ureteric stones on routine gynecological ultrasound examination in women presenting with pelvic pain. *Ultrasound Obstet Gynecol.* 2015;46:378–9.

25. Park SJ, Lim JW, Ko YT, Lee DH, Yoon Y, Oh JH, Lee HK, Huh CY. Diagnosis of pelvic congestion syndrome using transabdominal and transvaginal sonography. *AJR Am J Roentgenol.* 2004;182:683–8.

26. Gloviczki P, Comerota AJ, Dalsing MC et al. Society for Vascular Surgery; American Venous Forum. The care of patients with varicose veins and associated chronic venous diseases: Clinical practice guidelines of the Society for Vascular Surgery and the American Venous Forum. *J Vasc Surg.* 2011;53(Suppl 5):2S–48S.

27. Coakley FV, Varghese SL, Hricak H. CT and MRI of pelvic varices in women. *J Comput Assist Tomogr.* 1999;23:429–34.

28. Steenbeek MP, van der Vleuten CJM, Schultze Kool LJ, Nieboer TE. Noninvasive diagnostic tools for pelvic congestion syndrome: A systematic review. *Acta Obstet Gynecol Scand.* 2018;97:776–86.

29. Berton F, Gola G, Wilson SR. Perspective on the role of transrectal and transvaginal sonography of tumors of the rectum and anal canal. *AJR Am J Roentgenol.* 2008;190:1495–504.

30. Jansen E, Fransis S, Ahmad S, Timmerman D, Van Holsbeke C. Imaging in gynaecological disease: Clinical and ultrasound characteristics of mucocele of the appendix. A pictorial essay. *Facts Views Vis Obgyn.* 2013;5:209–12.

31. Miettinen M, Sarlomo-Rikala M, Lasota J. Gastrointestinal stromal tumors: Recent advances in understanding of their biology. *Am J Surg Pathol.* 1999;23:1109–18.

32. Teoh WC, Teo SY, Ong CL. Gastrointestinal stromal tumors presenting as gynecological masses: Usefulness of multidetector computed tomography. *Ultrasound Obstet Gynecol.* 2011;37:107–9.

33. Pinto V, Ingravallo G, Cicinelli E, Pintucci A, Sambati GS, Marinaccio M, D'Addario V. Gastrointestinal stromal tumors mimicking gynecological masses on ultrasound: A report of two cases. *Ultrasound Obstet Gynecol.* 2007;30:359–61.

34. Padmanaban N, Chandrabose PS, Esakki M, Kirubamani H, Srinivasan C. Gynaecological perspective of schwannoma: A rare pelvic tumour. *J Clin Diagn Res.* 2016;10:QD03–5.

35. Karaköse O, Pülat H, Oğuz S, Zihni İ, Özçelik KÇ, Yalta TD, Eken H. A giant ancient schwannoma mimicking an adnexal mass: Case report. *Medicine (Baltimore).* 2016;95:e4240.

36. Surendrababu NR, Cherian SR, Janakiraman R, Walter N. Large retroperitoneal schwannoma mimicking a cystic ovarian mass in a patient with Hansen's disease. *J Clin Ultrasound.* 2008;36:318–20.

37. Zikan M, Fischerova D, Pinkavova I, Slama J, Weinberger V, Dusek L, Cibula D. A prospective study examining the incidence of asymptomatic and symptomatic lymphoceles following lymphadenectomy in patients with gynecological cancer. *Gynecol Oncol.* 2015;137:291–8.

Index

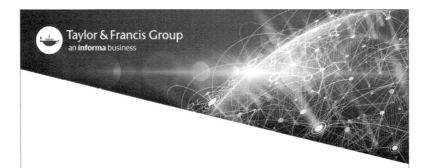